Broken Bonds
Surrogate Mothers Speak Out

Broken Bonds
Surrogate Mothers Speak Out

Edited by
Jennifer Lahl, Melinda Tankard Reist
and Renate Klein

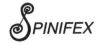

SPINIFEX

First published by Spinifex Press, 2019

Spinifex Press Pty Ltd
PO Box 5270, North Geelong, VIC, Australia 3215
PO Box 105, Mission Beach, QLD, Australia 3215
70-A Greenwich Ave #255, New York City, NY, USA 10011

women@spinifexpress.com.au
www.spinifexpress.com.au

Copying for educational purposes
Information in this book may be reproduced in whole or part for
study or training purposes, subject to acknowledgement of the
source and providing no commercial usage or sale of material occurs.
Where copies of part or whole of the book are made under part VB
of the Copyright At, the law requires that prescribed procedures be
followed. For information contact the Copyright Agency Limited.

Cover design by Deb Snibson, MAPG
In-house editing: Pauline Hopkins and Susan Hawthorne
Typeset in Utopia
Typeset by Helen Christie, Blue Wren Books
Printed by McPherson's Printing Group

A catalogue record for this
book is available from the
National Library of Australia

Paperback: 9781925581553
ePub: 9781925581584
Adobe PDF: 9781925581560
Kindle: 9781925581577

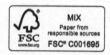

"[Surrogacy] is not only a desire to raise a child,
but also a demand that the mother be absent ..."
—Kajsa Ekis Ekman, *Being and Being Bought*

"For love is not to be bought, in any sense of the words ..."
—Mary Wollstonecraft, *A Vindication of the Rights of Woman*

Contents

Introduction

The Erased Women

In the 21st century, reproductive marketplaces are expanding globally. Renewed debate has taken place about the commercialisation and regulation of the baby-making industry. The public conversation has been captured by those with vested interests; doctors, IVF clinics, lawyers, counsellors and pro-surrogacy advocacy groups all want a piece of the lucrative pie.

But what happens to the voices of the other people involved; the so-called 'surrogate' mother, the egg 'donor', and the child that is grown in the birth mother's body from her own flesh and blood only to become a take-away baby and given to strangers who from now on are considered her or his parents?

'Surrogate' mothers[1] – without whom there would be no baby – are described as altruistic loving women who help to 'build' a family for desperate couples. To distance them from their child, they are reduced to 'carriers', 'ovens', and 'suitcases'. To make this heartless exploitation more palatable, surrogacy is promoted as a way for poor women to earn good money and support their families. *Time* magazine labelled pregnancy one of the '10 Best Chores to Outsource' (Lee-St John 2007). India's baby factories were "a big win for everyone involved," enthused *Forbes Magazine*. "You'd rent a

---

1 We are writing 'surrogate' mothers with inverted commas because we believe the use of 'surrogate' is a dehumanising description for a woman who gestates a child for nine months in her own body and gives birth to that child. We also use inverted commas for egg 'donation' as it is a dangerous medical procedure and cannot be compared to the ease with which sperm is harvested. Of course, the ease of sperm harvesting doesn't address the fact that children born of 'donor' sperm are still cut off from their biological beginnings.

1

nanny or a house painter. Why not rent a uterus?" the editorial asked (Smith 2013).

In *Broken Bonds: Surrogate Mothers Speak Out*, we challenge this dominant narrative around surrogacy and egg 'donation' and look behind the glitzy advertising and spin of third-party fertility brokers profiteering from the marketing of pregnancy and birth. We do this in the most compelling way possible – by bringing together the accounts of women – and one man who is the partner of a so-called surrogate mother – whose accounts disrupt the happy surrogacy stories.

These raw accounts expose the pro-surrogacy propaganda. They reveal the cruel disregard for the birth mother, the treatment of the child as a made-to-order commodity which has to be perfect or it will be rejected. The women's words invite us to also consider broader ramifications such as the mass factory farming of women (one surrogacy site identifies them by numbered code [2]) for their hair, breast milk, orifices and now wombs (Bindel 2016).

Broken Bonds asks us to consider surrogacy's problematic role in the dissection and eradication of biological motherhood. Kajsa Ekis Ekman, Swedish journalist, writer and activist, in *Being and Being Bought* (2013, p. 151) explains how a woman, once she has performed her 'service', must thereafter be absent.

> People who seek a surrogate have a very specific desire. It is not enough for them to get to know a child or to help to raise a child who is already alive ... No, it has to be their own genetic offspring, a newborn baby of whom the buyer has sole custody. This is always concealed in discussions about surrogacy – that it is not only a desire to raise a child, but also a demand that the mother be absent.

Surrogacy agencies and clinics love to display photographs of couples with babies born of surrogacy. Invariably, everybody is beaming with

---

2   Fourteen Vietnamese women were rescued from a surrogacy ring in Thailand. Some said they had been tricked, their visas confiscated, and officials believe some had been raped. The property was closely guarded 24 hours a day. Women were identified only by a numbered code (Thaivisa.com 2011).

happiness so that we should all feel delighted for them too; after all, a new baby is cause for celebration.

But in reality, these photos hide more than they reveal. Missing is the woman who carried and gave birth to the baby, the egg 'donor' who contributed half her genes, and perhaps even the sperm 'donor'. In addition, each individual involved in surrogacy is a member of family groups. They carry their own history, their kin and place, their memories and their secret hopes.

The aspiring parents may indeed have been on a difficult journey: multiple IVF failures with its physical and psychological suffering for the women.[3] Was it the nice surrogacy stories in glossy magazines that convinced them to continue their harrowing journeys of becoming parents? Had life without their 'own' children really become an impossibility to face?

We wonder how the beaming woman in the photo, holding the baby, arrived at the decision that another woman should grow and hand over a child for her. And still more perplexing is the question of what the commissioning male (or the two intending 'fathers') know of the profundity of pregnancy and birth. How do men expect a woman to give up a baby she grew in her own body?

> *I will pretend to the commissioning couple that I am so pleased I can make a baby for them. I will say that I love being pregnant and I really want to help. They will never know what I really feel … (Elena)[4]*

As for the baby, who can know what she has heard, felt, tasted and smelled before being given away to these new people? Despite her circumstances, she wants the breast milk and the warm skin of her mother, like all babies do. Will anybody tell her how she was made and transferred at birth, and at what cost?

---

3   The risks, commercialisation and poor outcomes of IVF are described and discussed by many commentators and experts; see for example Klein 2008 and Winston 2018.

4   These words are reminiscent of those in *Prostitution Narratives: Stories of Survival in the Sex Trade* (Norma and Tankard Reist, 2016) – women pretending to enjoy what is being done to them, to get through it and survive.

Relinquishing the baby soon after birth is the absolute worst ... I think the parents thought they were doing themselves a favor by not allowing me to hold her and comfort her ... People who engage in surrogacy are usually well-educated who know that the baby sees, hears, and smells its environment before she or he is born. And yet they are so willing to snatch it right away from its mother, give it another designation ... Babies aren't blank slates. (Michelle)

The 'surrogate' mother is usually not pictured in these family photos. The *whole point* is that she is not meant to be part of the new family. What was it that motivated her to undergo painful hormonal injections, the embryo transfer, the morning sickness, then to spend those nine months creating a baby in her body, only to give it away?

My first surrogacy journey should have been a huge red flag to me. But I didn't learn. I love being pregnant, I love excitement, I love people fussing over baby bellies and I love happy endings, you know ... I remain incredibly unwell and I have been diagnosed with post-traumatic stress disorder (PTSD). Two international couples have exploited me, lied to me, and have caused my family and me so much suffering. And all because I wanted to help them having a child in their lives. (Kelly)

We wonder what she was told, and by whom, about the surrogacy journey she would begin. Had she been informed that surrogacy is riskier to both herself and the baby than her own naturally conceived pregnancies? Babies born from surrogacy have higher rates of preterm birth and low birth weight, and 'surrogate' mothers have more obstetrical complications including gestational diabetes, hypertension and placenta previa. They often require antibiotics during the almost always obligatory caesarean section (Woo, Hindoyan, Landay *et al.* 2017).

When she signed the contract, who guided her through its contents, explaining the procedures and risks? How many tests, injections, hormonal drugs, scans, miscarriages, terminations, and procedures did she endure for this baby to grow in her womb? How did she feel about the developing baby and about the time when they would part? Did she heed the clinic's advice that this was not her child and had nothing to do with her? Did this requested separation of mind and body – in other words, dissociation – leave her feeling empty? Will she ever forget? The women in this book answer these questions and their answers are heart-breaking.

> *The pain never goes away. I am still an emotional basket case and struggle every day with this ... When I signed the paper, I thought I could do it. I did not realize it would break my heart. The pain and emptiness I feel have been unbearable.* (Cathy)

Surrogacy is the ultimate form of disconnection: the mother from her body; the body from her child; the child sold to people who have ordered their baby online via IVF clinics and brokers. These are the tools of neoliberal patriarchal capitalists.

Baby business empires and the myth of choice

The global surrogacy industry pockets around US$2.3bn each year (Cottingham 2017). But the 'surrogate' mother will only see a fraction of this money (some have ended up in worse debt) while the pockets of industry stakeholders (brokers, doctors, clinics and lawyers) are filled.

In *Misogyny Re-loaded*, Australian writer and feminist Abigail Bray (2013, p. 95) points out that women are ripe for exploitation in times of global economic recessions and downturns which often bring with them austerity measures including cutbacks in welfare: "As unemployment threatens an increasing number of women, exploitation has become preferable."

Long-time critic of reproductive technologies, Janice Raymond, also de-constructs the meaninglessness of 'choice' in such contexts:

> Choice occurs in the context of a society where, to put it mildly, there are fundamental differences of power between men and women. Yet feminists who oppose technological and contractual reproduction are vilified for supposedly claiming that "infertile women and, by implication, all women [are] incapable of rationally grounded and authentic choice" ... Little is said about why women are willing to submit

their bodies to the most invasive and harmful medical interventions – for example, because their lives are devalued without children, because of husband/family pressure, because there has been little research and few resources devoted to infertility, and because women are channelled into abusive technologies at any cost to themselves (Raymond 1996, p. 241).

And as Renate Klein explains in her 2017 book *Surrogacy: A Human Rights Violation*, women's 'choices' are in reality 'difficult decisions' that must be understood in the context of their emotional, spiritual, material, social and political lives.

The scaffolding of surrogacy is emotional and financial manipulation and, in many cases, outright deception. In commercial surrogacy, the manipulation takes the form of cash; almost all 'surrogate' mothers come from lower economic backgrounds and are often of different ethnicities and educational backgrounds than those of the intended parents. Sometimes the manipulation takes the form of appeals to compassion and kindness.

> *I am happy to have given life to these children and [I] have to give them [the children] away as a gift [to this couple] though my heart is hurting. These children are part of my life but the deal [the contract] was made right at the beginning and I have to keep it up by giving them away.* (Ujwala)

But even when there is no overt profit motive, we see in the accounts of so-called altruistic surrogate mothers that emotional manipulation and pressure can erode the true exercise of choice. Renate Klein's analysis of Australia's best known surrogacy case, in which Linda Kirkman gave birth to her child destined for sister Maggie, reveals the coercion that takes place within families and friendships (2017). Contributor Odette describes her own experience:

> *[The intended father] explained that further IVF was out of the question for Melanie because of her cancer. He said that he and Melanie had one frozen embryo that would only be viable for at most another two years. He asked me if I would be a surrogate for them using this one embryo. He explained that they both loved my hands-on parenting, my healthy*

lifestyle and diet, and my ability to teach Christopher right from wrong. They thought I was a perfect match as a surrogate for them. (Odette)

US 'surrogate' mother Kelly engaged in surrogacy three times to financially support her family when they were struggling from paycheck to paycheck. In the compelling 2018 film *#Big Fertility: It's all about the money,*[5] Kelly explains how she was hopeful each time, but instead she experienced stress, threats, dysfunctional intended parents, life-threatening illness, and outright betrayal. Today, she still struggles financially and can no longer have children. The film shows how a big industry was unscrupulous in exploiting a healthy young woman for profit. It also reveals the myriad holes in the argument that regulation and contracts can empower women when in reality the opposite is the case.

Liberal 'choice' feminists, for whom any decision a woman makes is a sign of freedom and empowerment, fail to analyse the conditions under which women exercise these so-called choices. The grief, loss, regret and powerlessness of the birth mothers is hidden under the façade of 'reproductive autonomy'. The 'surrogate' mother's 'right to bodily autonomy' conveniently aligns with the 'right' of another (wealthier) person to obtain a baby. We saw the ultimate expression of this in the case of a 28-year-old Japanese businessman, Mitsutoki Shigeta, who was granted custody of thirteen babies birthed by nine Thai surrogate mothers using multiple donor eggs. His wealth – emphasised by the judge – demonstrated again the feminisation of poverty and the way money is used to erase the mothers. None of the multiple egg 'donors' or 'surrogate' mothers will be part of their babies' lives. Media reports say Shigeta had previously raised other children from surrogacies in Cambodia and Japan (ABC News 2018). The court found 'for the happiness and opportunities the 13 children will receive from their biological father' they were 'the plaintiff's legal children' – the assumption being that his wealth (but not their birth mothers) is all they need for happiness (Hurst 2018).

---

5   CBC Network (2018). *#Big Fertility: It's All About the Money.* Watch at <https://vimeo.com/ondemand/bigfertility/289386333>

She is both raw material and factory

The 'gestational carrier', as they call her, is both raw material and factory. The baby is the 'product', made in and of the woman. Perhaps the intended parents provided the egg and sperm but often they do not, and another woman, the 'egg vendor', jeopardises her life and health for the harvesting of her eggs.

> ... *when fertility doctors see egg donors, they see anonymous women who represent tens of thousands of dollars to them. They care nothing for them. Donors are useful only until their eggs have been removed.* (Maggie)

Where there is a commercial trade in eggs, women can receive significant sums depending on how 'beautiful', 'intelligent' or 'accomplished' they are. Where it is illegal to buy human egg cells, some women 'donate' their eggs out of 'kindness' and are praised as 'angels' in the same way as 'surrogate' mothers are. Young women are aggressively courted and recruited with little or no mention of short- and long-term risks. And as with surrogacy, it's all about the money – not about women's wellbeing.

Maggie shares her heartbreaking story about multiple egg donations and now her terminal breast cancer diagnosis. "I went on to donate nine more times over ten years. ... I'd feel the warm glow of acceptance and mistakenly believed it meant I was loved. I never realized I was being used."

The woman who provides the egg is one part of the raw material. The body (and soul) of the 'surrogate' mother is the other. Without these women, there would not be an industry.

Quality control

While we hear a lot about 'love' being the driving motivation for all parties, it becomes clear that this 'love' is conditional on the end product being as 'perfect' as ordered. That's where quality control mechanisms such as prenatal testing, foetal reduction (terminating 'excess' foetuses) or abortion on grounds of 'disability' or 'wrong sex' enter the picture.

Sarah MacDonald (2014) lists some of the outcomes of surrogacy – which like other reproductive industry practices, has a strong base in eugenics.[6]

> There have been abortions ordered against a surrogate's religious beliefs. There have been female and male embryos destroyed because of gender (sic) selection. There have been eggs sold on the black market. Healthy foetuses have been terminated because proposed parents asked for multiple embryos to improve their chances ... and then ordered a 'reduction' ...

The Eastern European 'surrogate' mothers in *Broken Bonds* stated that if the baby was born with a disability, they would not get paid. What becomes of such babies, the women did not know.

Contributor Britni knows personally how easily dispensed with is a baby that doesn't meet quality-control orders:

> *For people that wanted a baby so badly, they were so quick just to dispose of these two 'imperfect' ones. But babies aren't disposable, they're humans and I was the one who felt life inside me. I'm the one that held the babies in my hands after I delivered them. They didn't realize what this did to me. I just don't think they deserve to be parents.* (Britni)

The destruction of the maternal bond

The resulting (flawless) baby is then expected to reciprocally love those who commissioned and paid for her, rather than the birth mother. The birth mother is counselled to *not* love the baby. But the baby is unaware of the deal.

After birth, the baby wants the mother in whose womb she has lived and whose voice, scent and rhythm has been her whole existence; she knows nothing else.

---

6   The eugenic base of reproductive technologies is explored in *Defiant Birth: Women Who Resist Medical Eugenics* (Tankard Reist ed. 2006).

In animal science, maternal separation is straightforwardly understood as one of the most stressful early adverse experiences in an animal's life (Récamier-Carballo *et al.*, 2017).

Even kittens and puppies must not be removed from their lactating mother before seven weeks of age.[7] Yet in adoption and surrogacy human babies can legally be separated from their lactating mother at birth, before the baby has even suckled. "The key to understanding the trauma of separation at birth is that, even when no longer physically connected, the mother and baby continue to be psychologically, emotionally and spiritually connected: this is the mother/baby dyad," writes Nancy Verrier in *The Primal Wound: Understanding the Adopted Child* (1996, p. 27).

Catherine Lynch, an adoptee, in a notable – and very personal – Submission to the Review of the Western Australian Surrogacy Act 2008 in Australia, writes (2018):

> During the 50s, 60s and 70s, now known as the 'baby-scoop era', thousands of us were removed from our gestational mothers for adoption. We are now adults and have important testimony to contribute to the debate about surrogacy.
>
> Those of us in the Stolen Generation and from the era of Forced Adoption have testified over and over again that the loss of our mothers is a devastating loss with profound life-long and intergenerational impacts. Is anyone even listening?
>
> Those of us who have suffered maternal-neonate separation testify that it has a life-long impact on our emotional and psychological wellbeing.

What does the surrogacy industry make of the evidence on maternal-child separation, the devastating loss, the life-long impacts?

One surrogacy website offers some heartbreaking suggestions. Their clinical social worker recommends that "throughout the process, the focus should be on the child's needs rather than the

---

7   For example, in Australia New South Wales Government (2009) and Victoria State Government (2018), under the provisions of the *Prevention of Cruelty to Animals Act 1986*.

intended parents' need to be parents ... That will result in a much better attachment and bonding process."

The process of what they call 'emotional transfer' is proposed for intended parents to develop healthy bonds with the new baby. Sending recordings of the intended parents' reading stories or their favourite music so the surrogate mother can play it to the unborn baby; having the birth mother sleep with a teddy then send it home with the baby to preserve her scent; placing the baby on the 'surrogate' mother's chest for some touch and smell ... and then handing the baby to the intended parents – complete strangers from the baby's perspective.

This social worker even suggests visiting the 'surrogate' mother in a couple of weeks: "It's just so reaffirming to the child that they haven't lost anyone, and it provides reassurance to everyone that the surrogacy process was successful," she says. And don't worry if the baby seems desperately unhappy: "Intended parents need to know that it's not related to the surrogacy or the transfer if the baby's fussy or upset" (Surrogate.com 2018).

Further examples of the totality of mother erasure can be seen in two articles which appeared in the same month.

In "'Who's the mother?': Two new dads embrace parenthood after surrogate birth"[8] published by CBC News, the commissioning male couple describe how the 'surrogate' Christine is "the person most often misidentified as the mother." (She is named on the child's birth certificate as mother, but that's because the laws are behind, the men say). Christine is praised for being "maternally detached" from the "entity growing inside of her" – a "super-power" which sets surrogates apart from other mere humans. "Hey Dads, you hold and support the Surrogates legs, cuz your baby is on its way," the young male doctor is quoted. At this point the mother doesn't even have a name. She is merely a *Surrogate* who needs her legs supported for the delivery of *their* baby. And then the mother-erasure climaxes

---

8   Joey Tremblay, CBC News, November 28, 2018 <https://www.cbc.ca/news/canada/saskatchewan/surrogate-new-dads-baby-born-regina-1.4922384>

with the newly born baby told "Don't fret baby. Not a single thing is missing. You do have a mother. You're looking at him ... We finally had a crystal clear answer. Who's the mother? Isn't it obvious? We are."

Baby Bette, of course, has no say.

At the same time over at *Good Men Project*, in what amounts to a large free ad for the surrogacy industry, the male author writes [9]: "Good candidates enjoy helping others and don't mind making small sacrifices to make a difference in the world ... Her ability to forego maternal attachment – and her 'small sacrifices' in pregnancy and birth, demonstrates she is 'emotionally stable'."

The message is that there's no need for a mother. Indeed what is required is that the mother is absent. This 'modern family' is founded on the destruction of the child's first family.

Kajsa Ekis Ekman summarised this well (2013, p.176):

> She must live for the child, think of the child in every daily action. Simultaneously, she must create distance between herself and her body, between herself and the child she bears – because a person must always make a distinction between what is her being and what is being bought. She must care about the child, but not get attached to it.

One anonymous woman wrote on a forum:

> I'm a few days away from giving birth to this baby. I love her way more than I planned. The thing is, I'm a surrogate. This selfless act is turning into the most selfish thoughts (Whitelocks 2016).

Denial of the rights of the child

Despite the commonly heard 'best interests of the child' mantra, in reality the rights of children born through surrogacy are utterly disregarded, explains Mirah Riben (2015):

---

9   'Five Ways to Know If You'd Make a Good Gestational Surrogate', Mian Azhar, November 30, 2018, <https://goodmenproject.com/parenting/five-ways-to-know-if-youd-make-a-good-gestational-surrogate/>

What, if any, rights or protection do the children of surrogacy have? Some who hire surrogates do so after being rejected as adopters because of age limits. Others fail or want to avoid a background check, which surrogacy does not require. Unlike adoption, surrogacy requires no home studies. Children can thus be ordered, paid for, and handed over to anyone, including pedophiles or others who may intend to mistreat them.

Donor conceived and adopted people have been speaking out for years about their sense of genetic bewilderment, and the pain of not knowing their biological origins.[10] Some groups representing child donors had success in changing laws so they can try to locate their genetic parents (though in many cases the change came too late and they discovered their medical histories were destroyed). However, in many countries the anonymity of gamete donors remains protected, thus preventing children from getting in touch. Think of how difficult it will be for a child born from a commercial surrogacy arrangement to trace their complex genetic and medical histories, with, for example, a 'surrogate' mother living in poverty in India, an egg 'donor' anonymously living in Ukraine, and possibly a sperm donor from Denmark. How will they find out their heritage and also their medical risk factors? What if their future love interest is actually their sibling?[11]

More fundamentally – do not children born through surrogacy arrangements have a right to a familial relationship with anyone that might be genetically connected to them, and to their birth mother who might have loved them and still loves them dearly?

'Surrogate' mothers who attempt to keep their babies because they fell in love with them, or suspected danger in the new family, meet with very strong resistance. Often, they are rendered powerless.

---

10 See Donor Conception Support Group of Australia Inc. 1997; Lorbach 2003.

11 A Dutch man in 2018 discovered he was conceived using donor sperm; after searching for his father, he found the donor was a 'super sperm donor' and he had at least 60 siblings in The Netherlands and possibly 1000 worldwide (du Cann and Petkar 2018).

Amongst the women in this collection, Toni was subject to racist abuse during her pregnancy and wanted to protect her baby from a home full of hate. She fought but lost the baby. Odette found out that the intended mother had threatened to kill herself as well as Odette at one point; she fought but is not even allowed to see her child. Cathy found the commissioning fathers to be lacking any compassion for her suffering and wondered how they could care for three tiny babies, but had to sign them away regardless.

'I would have asked for the children to be returned'

Surrogacy operates on the intellectual fiction that it does not matter who gestates a baby.

As the stories in this anthology show, the birth mothers often want to continue caring for the babies whom they have nurtured inside their bodies. They are at times taken by surprise about how strong this yearning is and how long it lasts.

> *In a way it is good that they are not in touch, otherwise I would have asked for the children to be returned.* (Sarala)

> I got attached ... it's ruined me. I don't know how to fix that. (Kelly, in *#Big Fertility*, CBC Network 2018)

In 1980, Elizabeth Kane became America's first commercial 'surrogate' mother. As she wrote herself, she 'carved the word *surrogate* into the American psyche' (Kane 1988, p. 271). When she had been an unmarried mother, she had given her newborn daughter up for adoption, For this reason she thought that she could manage surrogacy.[12]

Eight years later she wrote:

> I understand now that it was important to me to project an apple-pie image to the public. I had wanted to make surrogacy work so badly that I'd refused to let myself feel or think negatively about my decision to have

---

12 She is later re-united with daughter Heidi and acknowledges the suffering she endured as a result of both the adoption and the surrogacy.

Justin. Now that I have the freedom to look back, I know I should have talked about the emotional impact this pregnancy had on me and my family ... but I was incapable of speaking the truth ... My fears of being labelled a failure by the media or incurring the wrath of Justin's parents and Dr Levin silenced me. I still wanted to remain the perfect case ... I was plunged into depression – the type that was debilitating and marked by complete despair. I lived in a well of sorry so deep that not even my children could reach me (Kane 1988, p. 249).

In words that are wrenching to read, Kane asked, "How will I begin to explain to Justin that he was traded for the price of a new car? What will I say when he asks me why I never fought for him in court?" (Kane 1988, p. 265).

She now describes the experience as "nothing more than the transference of pain from one woman to another. One woman is in anguish because she cannot become a mother, and another woman may suffer for the rest of her life because she cannot know the child she bore for someone else" (Kane 1988, p. 272).

Commissioning parent Alex Kuczynski (2008) echoes Kane's assessment when she writes of cropping out the 'surrogate' mother's name in ultrasound photographs:

... I wanted her identity to disappear and mine to take its place.

As much as I tried to fight off the feeling, when I told others that I was expecting a baby – and this child was clearly not coming out of my womb – I would sometimes feel barren, decrepit, desexualized, as if I were branded with a scarlet "I" for "Infertile."

The impact on the remaining children is too often ignored or minimised. In *Birth Mother* (1988, pp. 253-257), Kane gives a heart-breaking depiction of the suffering and trauma of her children over the loss of their brother. Daughter Laura "covered her face with both hands and sobbed, 'I never got to hold my baby brother'." Her son Jeffrey would "look at pictures of babies and his little face would droop with sadness; "Baby's gone."

Birth mothers describe their devastation at not being allowed to hold their child before saying goodbye, or being permitted only a fleeting cuddle, sobbing as they hand their child back. Sherrie, who gave birth to a child for her sister puts it like this:

> I can't describe the depth of sadness I felt when I came home without the child I loved, carried within me, and gave birth to. It was as if I had a child die ... I just couldn't help but love this child like my own, because it was my own ... As I watched their car driving away that day on the gravel road, I felt like the dust left behind to scatter in the corn fields (in Ekis Ekman 2013, p. 187).

The stories in *Broken Bonds* echo the sentiments of early 'traditional' surrogacy cases of bonding, attachment and longing for the child. Another woman, Laschelle Baker, changed her mind the third time she acted as a 'surrogate' mother, unable to hand over the twins she gave birth to in 2009. Judgement was swift. As documented by Ekman (2013, pp. 188-190) she was called a demon, a witch, just evil, worse than a whore and (bizarrely) 'baby-selling hoe.' Non-compliant birth mothers are seen as 'shameful.' They have stepped out of their place as an invisible 'gestational carrier': no longer acquiescent, no longer obedient, no longer submissive.

Unbearable pain. Unbearable emptiness.

Contributor Britni, after her loss, is seeing a psychiatrist and taking anti-depressants and anti-anxiety medications, along with birth control medication to regulate her hormones due to stress and irregular bleeding.

Marie Anne now has PTSD and postpartum psychosis, including severe mood swings, depression, suicidal thoughts, anxiety and daily panic attacks. She deeply regrets her surrogacy and writes with the purpose of dissuading anyone else from doing it.

'Altruistic surrogate' Odette comments:

> *I am so sad about what has happened with this surrogacy — but also angry. I feel betrayed, hurt, and I am still suffering mentally and physically from what I have been through. I have great trouble sleeping. Not a day goes by that I do not regret handing over Mitchell ... I regret not fighting for*

him after his birth. Not a day goes by where I do not think about him and wonder if he is safe.

The baby's new legal and social arrangement is constructed out of the wreckage of his or her biologically embodied reality. The 'modern family' created by surrogacy triumphs at the cost of the mother-child dyad. Its destruction leaves permanent deep wounds on both.

Our contributors – to whom we are deeply indebted for trusting us with their painful memories – live in the USA, the UK, Canada, India, Australia, Russia, Romania, Georgia and Hungary. Initially they were trying to help, to change someone's grief to joy, or to simply make financial ends meet. Invariably, they are cut off from the child(ren) they gave birth to. And often, they are left sick, physically and emotionally.

Like any woman who has carried and birthed a child, pregnancy and birth has changed them. Surrogacy remains unfinished business. The women struggle with unresolved grief, many remaining bitter about the deceits and lies they suffered. They try to heal from the trauma, to come to terms with loss. Some are still fighting in the courts. Some know they will likely never again see the child they held so briefly at birth. All are courageously speaking out in the hope that others like them will not be fodder for the global surrogacy industry.

As Michelle puts it:

I would never, ever advise other women to carry a baby for someone else, whether genetically related or not. Whatever they promise you will not come to fruition. I don't see how a woman can carry a baby and not want to hold it, not want to breastfeed it, not want to change its diapers and whisper loving words in its ear.

It doesn't matter what are the child's origin, the woman who carried the child has ties to it. To pretend otherwise is just ignorance. You will be hurt. I suggest to every woman who thinks about becoming a surrogate: please consider another way, whether it's for the money, or the delusional idea of self-fulfillment, or whatever. You're not just hurting yourself, you're hurting the baby you carry inside you as well.

It was challenging for our contributors to share their experiences. Surrogacy (and egg 'donor') contracts often include a clause requiring confidentiality, effectively silencing the parties. And the internet does not welcome stories from the dark side of surrogacy – it unsettles the narrative of happy families and selfless angels.

We challenge these attempted justifications of baby trading. The world needs to listen to women's experiences, even when painful and inconvenient.

> *Every time I share this story, it gets just a little easier. Shame silences. I get to reclaim my voice and my spirit a bit more each time I talk about my experience. I know there are people who think I deserve what happened to me. Many have told me exactly that. I don't share this story for those people. I share my story and what happened to me – from the decisions I made to the end result – because I hope something good will come from the living nightmare I went through.* (Maggie)

We believe that as feminists we must honour women's stories and then act to bring about needed change. We see *Broken Bonds* as a classic form of collective action. We hope you will be as moved as we have been by these desolating accounts. *We are determined to see all forms of surrogacy abolished.* Our Afterword describes the global resistance against this industry.

Jennifer Lahl
Melinda Tankard Reist
Renate Klein

Signing the Paper in Blood
Cathy (Canada)

I heard about surrogacy through the internet. I even joined a support group for surrogate mothers. Being a member of this group was very addictive and they became like family to me. Every day I would read about their embryo transfers and pregnancy tests. It was exciting to be a part of the group. There were no sad stories ever mentioned. Everyone was happy and upbeat. I couldn't wait to get started being a surrogate mother and help build a family!

Finally after speaking on the phone with a couple a few times we were matched! I decided I was going to help a gay couple because I could still be their only mom – the children would always have a mom and I would be that person.

The couple seemed nice, and we were supposed to meet in person but they never seemed to have the time. Even though we all lived in Canada we still were not close geographically. So, we just spoke on the phone and connected that way.

When we signed our contract, we still had not met and this was about a year after we had first spoken. I felt they were always very busy. One of the men lived about ten hours away and the other was working overseas in Mexico. So, we just kept moving forward with our plans. I had my psychiatric evaluation, which I passed, but to be honest, I should not have passed it. I had suffered a miscarriage with my own child while I had been waiting to start the surrogacy process and I was still very upset about this. I also had issues with my adoptive mom that I have always ignored, and I really should have dealt with, but since I had already agreed to help, I told myself I could wait until after the surrogacy. Then I would have another baby of my own and deal with these issues between me and my adoptive mother.

Things went very slowly because the couple kept having problems and dragging the whole process out. They had previously chosen another surrogate who was a friend and who backed out of the arrangement. Then their egg donor, who was also a friend of theirs, backed out because she supposedly didn't want to travel to Mexico to do the egg retrieval process.

The intended parents were going to use a clinic in Mexico because they wanted to do sex selection, which is prohibited in Canada, but the Mexican clinic would provide it. I was a bit worried about going outside of Canada to Mexico because you hear about medical problems in foreign countries and I had never been to Mexico, but they assured me it would all be fine.

They ended up using an anonymous egg donor they found in Mexico, but even that was full of problems as it took months and months to sort out the egg donor issues and to synchronise our cycles. All these problems caused the whole process to drag on and looking back now, these should have been red flags for me.

But I ignored all these setbacks because I figured all these problems weren't that bad. I thought I was just being silly and worrying about nothing and I told myself it was all going to be fine.

When I arrived in Mexico I finally met the couple for the first time. They seemed ok to me, but my friend who went with me just didn't like them – he said they seemed too needy. But I thought they were just stressed and were overly concerned with trying to make a good first impression on me.

They decided to use sperm from only one of them and at the last minute they decided against the sex selection. The plan was to perform a transfer of two five-day-old embryos. I was in Mexico for only a single day for the whole process!

I went home and waited to do home pregnancy tests. My pregnancy test was positive at four days post transfer. I was so excited! I told the surrogacy support group all about it and oh boy it was so exciting! I told the couple but it was strange because they did not seem excited at all. They were very blunt, saying that they would wait for blood tests to confirm that I was in fact pregnant. My blood test numbers were through the roof and again I was so excited, but the couple still was not excited, they were just matter of fact. They acted like I was mailing them a package and responded with "Ok, that's great – keep us posted."

Finally, at 14 days after a positive pregnancy test, it came time for my ultrasound. All went well and the ultrasound showed that I was pregnant with twins! I was so excited but again, the couple still showed no real interest in the news of the pregnancy. I received very few phone calls from them and they didn't come to any ultrasounds. I have no idea why they didn't come as I always told them well in advance of the appointments so that they could arrange their schedules to be there. My understanding is that most intended parents want to come to at least one of the appointments with the surrogate.

Two weeks later, I went for another ultrasound and once again they didn't come. This ultrasound was a complete and utter shock because they found a third baby! I now was told I was carrying triplets at ten weeks into the pregnancy. The bigger shock was that the babies were not identical, meaning that the clinic had messed up and implanted me with three embryos and not the two we had agreed on. I almost fell off the table. I called the couple and not only were they not excited but they blamed me for being pregnant with triplets. They told me that one of the babies must not even be theirs! I was in shock and disbelief about how cruel they were to me. Little did I know this was only the beginning of what was going to be a very bad situation.

The people I was supposed to have the children for were cold and unfeeling and treated me with little compassion. They never came with me to any doctor's appointment or ultrasound, or expressed any interest in my health and well-being. To them, I might as well have been a cow or a dog. I was not treated as a person. They were not there physically or emotionally for me.

The pregnancy was not easy on my physical health either. I was 46 years old at the time and had a two-year-old of my own as well as two young adult daughters. I was on hospital bed rest for two months during my 7th and 8th months of the pregnancy.

I developed gestational diabetes as well as pre-eclampsia, mostly due to my age and the high-risk pregnancy of carrying triplets. I was put into a medical coma for about a day into my last month of the pregnancy just to save my life.

The couple called the doctor, for the first time ever, four days before the delivery and announced to the doctor that this was a surrogate pregnancy and they were the parents of the babies, not me.

I was rushed in for an emergency cesarean section at 33 weeks. I had developed a heart problem that caused a lot of difficulty and made it hard to control my blood pressure.

I gave birth to three beautiful baby girls. They were born early at about 33 weeks and because of their birth weights – they weighed 1.5, 2.5 and 3 pounds – they needed to be in a neonatal intensive care unit for about three months. One was very sick and had to have surgery for necrotizing enterocolitis (NEC), which is a common bowel problem in premature infants. I was not allowed to hold my children, I couldn't visit them, and I wasn't even allowed to know how they were doing. I could not tell them that Mommy loved them. I was not there to see their first smiles, or hear their first coos. I was devastated by this and still am.

For the 24 hours after giving birth, I fought for my life. I was on a ventilator. My blood pressure was still all over the place. People were having me sign documents when I was so very groggy – papers allowing the intended fathers visitation in the nursery, and I signed away my parental rights relinquishing the babies during this state. I was still groggy and not really able to understand what was happening and I shouldn't have been asked to sign such important papers. My friend even had to sign some documents because I was unable to.

The couple I had the babies for came to see me and my daughters in the hospital. My oldest daughter, aged 23 at the time, explained to them I almost died. Their response was, "Well, she knew what it was going to be like being a surrogate!" They showed no compassion at all for me and the fact that I almost died, and my children almost lost their mother.

When I told them I was in pain post-op as I lost my uterus after delivery, one of the fathers was telling me about his hernia surgery and how painful that had been for him.

How could a couple that was so cruel and lacking in compassion be the same people that were going to raise three tiny fragile babies? I was devastated because of their total lack of concern for me and my children.

There was nothing as a surrogate mother that I could do legally to change the situation. If you are going to give your child up for adoption, you can change your mind, but for me there was no way out. It was like I had signed the paper in blood and there was no un-doing this. I had wanted out of the contract when I was four months pregnant but I had no legal help. The lawyer that was supposed to be my lawyer didn't represent my interests. Since the couple had paid her, she said there was a conflict of interest and her interests were with the intended parents. Yet it wasn't a conflict before when she was explaining the contract and having me sign it. I was told there was nothing I could do. Apart from having an abortion and killing three innocent babies, which I could not do, I was stuck.

My children were bought and the law said it was ok. I was given $20,000 Canadian dollars for reimbursed expenses related to the pregnancy and this is how Canada gets away with so-called altruistic surrogacy.

It has been two years since I have seen my daughters, even though they live only an hour away. The pain never goes away. I am still an emotional basket case and struggle every day with this.

I have missed seeing them learn to crawl and walk. I missed their first birthday and first words all because I signed a paper agreeing that the babies were not mine. When I signed the paper, I thought I could do it. I did not realize it would break my heart. The pain and emptiness I feel have been unbearable.

The Biggest Mistake of My Life
Oxana (Georgia)
As told to Eva Maria Bachinger[1]

My mother looks after my son. I won't see him for four months. He has his own view: that what is in my tummy is not his sister. He also does not want that this child looks anything like him. He thinks I am a kind of vessel, or actually, a sort of rocket carrier.

My pregnancy is supervised by an agency in Georgia, but it is me who is solely responsible for the baby. If the child is ill, I have to return the money for the tests I had. If it is born with a disability, they will not pay me any money. In this way, there are no risks for the agency, and none at all for the commissioning parents or parent. I don't know mine; he is a single man from Denmark. He has only seen a photo of me. I do hope that the child will have a good life, that it gets everything I can't give it. I am worried that my connection to the child is stronger than I thought. In fact, I feel sick in my stomach when I think about handing over this child. But there is nothing I can do. I just hope it happens fast.

When the girl is born, the father does not arrive. He does not turn up for five weeks.

Now that the baby is here, I have totally fallen in love with her. But I have to give her away. This is a terrible time for me. The surrogacy was the biggest mistake of my life. I thought I could do it. I will never ever do this again.

---

1   I conducted this interview for my 2015 book *Kind auf Bestellung. Ein Plädoyer für klare Grenzen* [Child to Order: A Plea for Clear Boundaries], Deutike Verlag, Vienna. Sentences in italics are my comments. Translation by Renate Klein.

Anonymous No More:
How I Was Groomed to Be a Multiple Egg Donor
Maggie (USA)

Every time I share this story, it gets a little easier. Shame silences. I get to reclaim my voice and my spirit a bit more each time I talk about my experience. I know there are people who think I deserve what happened to me. Many have told me exactly that. I don't share this story for those people. I share my story and what happened to me – from the decisions I made to the end result – because I hope something good will come from the living nightmare I went through.

I have people in my life now who love and support me. I have cheerleaders and their cheers roar louder than any of the people I care nothing about who continue to try to silence this story with accusations and shame. What was done to me reflects poorly on the doctors, nurses, the counselor, and all the others involved who claimed to represent my best interests. Health professionals who took an oath to keep their patients safe and do no harm. It does not reflect poorly on me. I never took advantage of a young woman's altruistic nature and naïveté.

The hurt, anger, fear, and blame I once felt have subsided. All that remains now is a desire to educate, a drive to have my story be the foundation for change. Let this story serve as a message of hope and encourage others to see women as more than baby-making commodities.

In 2002, I met a woman through a friend at a party. I was there supervising the toddler-aged children until they went to bed. The woman was a nurse at a fertility clinic. I was 21, she was in her early

40s. She spent some time asking me about my interests. Nothing strange. It seemed like she was just wanting to get to know me. In a relatively short time, this woman knew I liked kids, was a struggling college student working several part-time jobs and still taking out loans. I'm sure she could tell I was naïve, sheltered, and insecure. Anyone who spent two minutes with me then would have noticed those traits about me. Here was a woman who had just met me and she was telling me I was beautiful, intelligent, capable, and had a lot going for me. She wasn't wrong. Those things were true. They still are. The difference then was my perception of my self-worth. I was struggling with depression, felt awkward in my body, was silently confused about my sexuality, and desperately wanted to be liked and fit in. In many ways, I wasn't that different from other young women my age. My biggest flaw was a desire for others to like me and my need to be seen as a good person. I'd do almost anything to prove this. I craved hearing that I was liked, that I was kind and generous, and that I made others happy. I could quite easily be talked into doing things for others with just a little praise. That is where I believed my value was: in what I was able to do for others.

The nurse kept complimenting me that night. The way I carried myself, my intelligence and independence. My belief in women's rights and desire to be a respected feminist. At some point during the party, after grooming me all evening, she pulled me aside and suggested I think about donating my eggs. She said people would pay a lot of money for my eggs and again showered me in compliments. I said I wasn't interested in doing it just for the money. Her response was that the money could go towards paying my student loans and I'd be in a better place when I graduated. That did appeal to me. Making a smart decision to get further ahead, faster. Pay off debt and not have any ties or owe anyone. And I wasn't using my eggs right now. I didn't think I would ever want to have kids. Why not donate my eggs to someone who couldn't get pregnant on their own? After all, that would be really generous, kind, and would definitely make someone happy. I began to think about it. I asked what the risks were. Virtually none, she said. Just some discomfort and a big time commitment. So I made an appointment to go to the clinic and meet with her.

I did my research before going in. It was 2002. I googled egg donation. All that came up were advertisements recruiting donors. 21-year-old me did not understand how the design of the language, images, and concepts in these advertisements was incredibly calculated: "Be an angel, make their dreams come true." Beautiful young women, beaming with sunlight on their faces, presumably having donated their eggs and in doing so, finding eternal bliss. There was nothing stated about risks; no studies showing donors having adverse effects. So I went to the appointment and it was more of the same. If I did this, if I donated my eggs, I would be loved, respected, chosen as beautiful and intelligent, seen as kind and generous. On top of all that, they were going to pay me to do it. And the worst that could happen was that I'd have a little tummy bloating and discomfort. So I made the decision to just start the process. Fill out the paperwork, take the tests. My information would go in a donor file and maybe one day, someone might see it and choose me.

That day came very quickly. Within weeks, I got a call from the nurse who breathlessly told me I had been chosen by a lovely couple and she knew we were a perfect match. The nurse knew exactly what she was doing. It never occurred to me that I could still say no. That option was never offered. The momentum of the process was so fast I didn't have time to think about it. Although I hadn't committed to or signed any agreements, I was treated as though I had. Language changed subtly and they started to refer to me as 'the donor'. I felt stuck. I just wanted everyone to be happy.

There was paperwork I needed to sign. Written out plain as day, right in front of me, were forms declaring there were no side effects or known complications for the procedure. I had to give myself shots of hormones to prepare my body to donate. The drugs originally came in two small vials. I had to use syringes to mix them, then draw in the correct amount into a new syringe before I could give myself an injection. When you go to a pharmacy and pick up a prescription, it comes with warnings about interactions, side effects and risks. Yet here was a doctor in a doctor's office handing me pills and vials, which were labeled but with no additional information or warnings. So I trusted them. They were healthcare providers and professionals. I had no reason not to. They loved me. I wouldn't figure out for another ten years that when fertility doctors see egg donors, they see anonymous women who represent tens of thousands of dollars to them. They care nothing for them. Donors are useful only until their eggs have been removed. Then they can be discarded like trash. That's the danger of being anonymous. To the doctor, you're someone who is going away once you've been used and paid. To the recipient, you're a nameless photo in a binder of profiles of women.

And who writes the profile? It's a combination of the donor recruiter and the donor. The donor recruiter is a non-medical professional in the office that handles processing paperwork, interviewing donors, scheduling physicals and psychological evaluations, and they take photos and build profiles. They are responsible for getting donors to commit to donating. I filled out a pack asking me questions about my likes, interests, and hobbies. Books I enjoyed, food I liked, my ethnic heritage. On paper I looked good. I could be whatever I told them I wanted to be. Recipients saw a profile of a young Caucasian female, dark hair and eyes, thin and fit, athletic, soft spoken, an academic, and someone with multiple and varied interests. Somehow, my years of failed treatments for depression and anxiety didn't make it in the profile. Those were about the worst things I had going at that point. I had some suicidal thoughts, but nothing more than the average college student. I later heard stories of donors who hid drug addictions, family history of diseases, and domestic abuse.

I completed my first donor cycle. As I woke up in the recovery room after the retrieval, that same nurse was there. "You lit up like the Christmas tree in Times Square! I can't wait to use you as a donor again," she said. I will never forget her words. In that moment

I thought of myself, "You did something worthy of praise. They're proud of you and thankful to you." Now, all I can think of when I remember her words is that she was honest. She couldn't wait to 'use' me again.

It was as though completing one donor cycle somehow meant I'd be willing to continue, even though I'd never agreed to be a multiple donor. It was expected. And again I felt stuck. Like I couldn't say no. If I did, I'd be letting these people down and they were counting on me. Women couldn't fulfill their dreams of motherhood without me. I was needed.

I went on to donate nine more times over ten years. I didn't let myself go to a place of questioning it. I just fell into a routine of them calling me, excitedly telling me I was chosen. I'd feel the warm glow of acceptance and mistakenly believe it meant I was loved. I never realized I was being used.

Each time I went through the process, it would be slightly different than the previous time. The brand of birth control pills changed. The hormone injections began coming in pre-filled syringes where you screwed the needle in and dialed in the dosage. I once became so uncomfortable during a retrieval, the doctor started knocking me out completely on subsequent donations so I wouldn't feel anything. After every donation my ovaries, which were normally the size of a walnut, would swell. The worst it ever was, they swelled to the size of a grapefruit. I'd waddle around like I was five months pregnant, my stomach distended from enlarged ovaries, and they would reassure me everything was fine and this was completely normal. Within a month, the swelling would decrease and my ovaries would eventually return to walnut size. During the time they were swollen, everything was sensitive to the touch. I'd wear baggy clothes so no one would ask questions, furthering the feelings of shame and the belief that although I was doing this great act and helping others, I wouldn't be accepted by the outside world and my friends and family who would never understand. I had to be anonymous, and I had to hide what I was doing.

Several interactions reinforced the need to keep the fact I was donating a secret – reminding me I must remain anonymous. When I was in college, I lost a couple of friends when I told them I was donating. They were religious and accused me of playing God. One of them told me if a couple couldn't get pregnant on their own, it was a message from God they should not be parents. I found this belief so abhorrent it made me even more certain I was doing the right thing. I also confided in a boyfriend who immediately broke up with me and a family member who then accused me of selling their unborn biological relations. Each interaction was confusing and hurtful, and I turned to the nurses at the clinic for guidance in how to respond. They would reassure me that not everyone was strong enough to do what I was doing, that I was special and I was giving the greatest gift. And so I continued to donate every time they called me.

Then I found myself, at 31, divorced, crying at the fertility doctor's office about my marriage falling apart, losing my home and feeling extremely depressed. The doctor told me he'd use me as a donor again, get me some money, and since I was working as a communications officer in a police dispatch center, I could just move on with my life and meet a nice police officer. Here is what should have happened in that moment. A doctor who really cared about their patient would and should have said, "I can tell this is a difficult time for you. Anyone would be struggling. Now is not the time for you to be making a serious decision like donating your eggs again. See a counselor and work through the depression." But a fertility doctor doesn't see donors as patients or people. Recipients are the paying clients. Donors are just little egg incubators. Just anonymous bodies producing eggs like children making shoes in a sweatshop. Once the shoe is made, you take it, shut the door so you don't have to look at who made it, and put it on the shelf and sell it for thousands. You do it enough, you don't see the faces anymore. You just see dollar signs.

That's what still stings a little. At some point throughout all this, the fertility doctor, whom I trusted and mistakenly believed liked me, made a decision that risking my health and well-being was worth some amount of money. I was a commodity.

I donated that tenth time and it felt different from every time before. A nurse at the clinic began to talk to me throughout the process and said she thought the doctor was doing some shady things. She didn't say what exactly. But she'd come in and do my ultrasounds and I'd be lying there, crying and depressed. She'd say, "You know, he always gets so many eggs from you. You should demand more money. He has money so he should give it to you." It made the transaction seem tainted in some way. I didn't feel like I was doing it that time for the good that might come from it. It felt desperate. It felt dark and sleazy. I couldn't bring myself to feel any comfort or glow from their compliments. My life was falling apart and I didn't see a future. I no longer knew who I was.

Shortly after that last donation, I felt a lump in my breast. I fixated on it for months. I told myself it was nothing, but as I watched it grow in size the more I obsessed over it. I finally went to my primary care physician (PCP). She sent me for a mammogram. They told me it was nothing. You're too young and have no risk factors for breast cancer they said. Yet the lump grew. I went back to my PCP a while later and told her I was really getting worried about it. She sent me for another mammogram and an ultrasound. I was told again that there was nothing there. My PCP and I weren't comfortable with that result. She sent me to a breast surgeon for a biopsy. The breast surgeon did a punch biopsy, which to this day remains the worst physical pain I have ever felt. She took a hollow needle and placed it over the lump, which in my case was on the side of my nipple. The needle is pushed into the skin and the lump to remove a portion for a biopsy. Twenty-four hours later she was telling me I had breast cancer. Another week later and she was telling me I had stage four estrogen positive metastatic invasive ductal carcinoma. Breast cancer that had spread to my bones and my liver. Terminal cancer.

I called my friends and family. Everyone I told had the same question. How? How do you have terminal breast cancer at 32? I was healthy. Depressed, but physically healthy. I was careful about what I ate, I worked out, I rarely drank alcohol, I didn't use drugs or smoke cigarettes. I was good to my body. Why would it revolt in this way? How had cancer come in and spread this far this quickly?

My family and friends suspected being an egg donor had played a role. I was unwilling to believe it. I refuted their points saying, "No, these were doctors. They had to inform me about risks and they assured me there were none. They can't just lie to patients." Except fertility doctors aren't really doctors in the sense of what we expect from a physician who is treating us for the flu, or allergies, or even cancer. A fertility doctor is someone whose industry is largely unregulated. Even now, the only real 'recommendation' is a suggestion that fertility doctors not use a donor more than six times. No one is there to stop them though. Egg donors are presented with the claim there are no risks, not because studies on egg donation and donors have proven this, but because donors are an anonymous population that has never been medically tracked or studied. So there are no directly proven risks that indicate links between egg donors and cancers.

All that exists now is anecdotal evidence from the brave donors who come forward amid all the shaming and slander to share their stories as young women with debilitating and severe diseases, cancers, strokes, and their own fertility issues. "So what?" People say, "It's just a few women. That's not enough to come to any conclusive result." Well, there are more women with similar stories who have filed lawsuits, settled, and signed non-disclosure agreements. There are women who have died before they could share their story. And there are women who can never come forward because they donated anonymously. Because someone they know did not approve of it – and they are silenced by the shame of what has happened to them: to their body, their health, and to their life. Women who were healthy, fit, intelligent, and dreaming of bright futures. And they have one more thing in common. They decided to donate their eggs.

It took me just over a decade to finally believe it, but with the encouragement and support of strong and dedicated women and with hard work and personal growth on my part, a light was finally shining on the abusive and shameful scheme I fell for at 21. And here I am now, 16 years after my first donation, living with terminal cancer. It's a cancer that normally afflicts post-menopausal women who have had children. I was nowhere close to menopause and have no children. The only way my oncologist and treatment team could surmise any treatment being effective was to place me in menopause. So at 32, I had a complete hysterectomy. My body hasn't felt like it's been mine for almost half my life. I've only just begun, four years post chemotherapy treatments, to love my body as it is. When the nurse and the doctor lied to me and conned me into becoming an egg donor, they stole parts of my life. I will never be pregnant or give birth. I spent years of my life in treatment and missed out on many experiences during that time. I lost my ovaries and uterus and my body no longer responds the same way sexually. I meet people I think I might be interested in dating and instead of just having to share that I donated my eggs a few times, I have to disclose a terminal cancer diagnosis and all the baggage that comes with it. All because I let someone use me.

Once They Found out I Didn't Have the Perfect Baby, I Was Disposable
Britni (USA)

I have four children and I feel so blessed to be a mother. I have a few friends who have struggled to get pregnant, and friends that have lost pregnancies and babies, so that kind of just struck something within my heart. When I was done having kids, I wanted to reach out and help.

I saw an ad to be an egg donor or a surrogate, and originally I signed up to be an egg donor. But as a nurse I kind of know how they do surrogacy and how the whole process works. So I decided to do that instead.

Money was a small factor in the decision. I knew there was compensation for taking part and that it was substantially more for surrogacy than for egg donation. I probably wouldn't have done it for free, not for someone that I didn't know. If it were someone close to me, I probably would have done it just for enough money to cover my medical costs, and to cover time off work, something like that, but for a stranger, no.

When I signed up with the agency, the woman who did my egg donation profile was starting her own company, and she had intended parents in mind that she wanted to match me with personally. So she reached out and asked if I would consider being a surrogate for them. It was something I had to decide – whether I could actually do that and have a baby and give it up. After knowing how badly the couple wanted a baby and knowing in my heart I was done having a family,

I thought, yes, I could do this for them. So that's what brought me to this decision.

The original agency branch was in Chicago but the agency person in Michigan was the one who reached out in my area and the intended parents were also out of state.

I talked on the phone with the intended parents about what kind of things we expected, and then we did a Skype call, and then we did meet in person when I did all my screening with the doctors. The intended parents offered to pay me $30,000 for a single pregnancy, or $40,000 if it were twins. We signed a contract.

They used a donor egg and donor sperm, so genetically it was not their child. I know that the husband is not infertile – he has a 12-year-old from a previous marriage, but he was older, he was 50. The wife had prior cancer, so she couldn't use her own eggs, as the medication she was on can cause birth defects. They just wanted a chance of better genetics, so that's why they used donor sperm as well as donor eggs.

I actually agreed to have two embryos transferred and carry twins, however during the thawing of the frozen embryos, one did not survive. The doctors thought the remaining embryo was multiplying fast, and made us make a quick decision to just do the one, so we transferred just one embryo.

I got pregnant on the first try. The intended mother came down for my six-week ultrasound, and the agency person came down as well. That was kind of a bonding moment and we saw the heart beat for the first time. As a precaution, they wanted me to do a 12-week ultrasound just to make sure the baby was developing fine, because of the risks with IVF.

At the 12-week ultrasound we found out that the embryo had split, and I was actually carrying identical twins. However, they were conjoined at the abdomen. This was November 2017. This was a big bombshell that we now had to deal with.

There was an 'abortion clause' in the contract: I had agreed to terminate the pregnancy if there were disabilities.

The doctors said the best-case scenario for this type of twins is that usually they share a liver and abdomen, or a liver and bowel, which can be separated, and it looked hopeful, as long as they developed normally.

The intended parents took four days to think about it and then told me to abort.

I was in shock. This type of abnormality is incredibly rare, and for it to happen to me ... I had been just so hopeful. I thought the intended parents would want to continue the pregnancy, because we didn't know all the answers yet. I sought second medical opinions, including from a high risk perinatologist. I was told that these babies could have a normal and healthy life. The doctors recommended that I should get more testing done at 18 weeks, and meet with the surgical team.

I knew in my heart that I wasn't going to terminate the pregnancy. I was just taking time to explore all my options, both medically and legally. I sought out lawyers who looked over my contract, and sought out opinions from other doctors.

During this time, I did not feel at all supported by the agency. The agency person was acting on behalf of the intended parents. She said, "Britni, they don't want to have babies with deficits, they don't want to have issues or babies that have to go through surgery. She goes, "My son has autism, it is so hard for me, you have to understand where they are coming from." She was really on their side with abortion.

It was awful because I put my body through so much for them, I was willing to have a high-risk pregnancy for them, and time away from work and my children, and I felt like once they found out I didn't have the perfect baby, I was disposable.

Unfortunately, at 14 weeks, with my follow up ultrasound, they saw that the babies no longer had heartbeats. I was devastated because at that point I felt like everything was going right: the lawyers gave me good news, the doctors were still hopeful and I was hoping to fight the contract and maybe even keep the babies.

So when I found out there was no heartbeat, it was my loss as the surrogate mother, not the intended parents.'

The next day, the doctors induced labor and the babies were delivered naturally without a D & C. They were boys.

The intended parents and the agency have not tried to contact me once since this happened. They have not inquired after my welfare at all. The monthly payments stopped immediately.

Thinking about my decision to be a surrogate since that time, I definitely should have researched more. Once you decide to be a surrogate, you hear all these amazing good stories and you never think to research the bad ones; you never think to ask what could go wrong, and if it does go wrong, is the contract in my favor? What I experienced was that when things went wrong, nothing was in my favor. I was the one affected, physically and mentally, I was the one locked into a contract; it was devastating.

I think the doctors connected with the agency should have gone into more detail. They did say, "oh yeah, you could have a loss," but they did not sit down and go over scenarios, and explain how it would affect me and how that is reflected in the contract. I think they should discuss it in more detail when you are agreeing to something this major.

I don't think I would ever consider surrogacy again. It was too hard for me emotionally to go through that loss. One of the reasons I did it was because of the women who have experienced losses, and I couldn't imagine that. But now that I know the loss myself, I couldn't go through the sort of physical and emotional stuff I went through again.

All my children knew about the babies and I think they were as invested as I was, talking about the babies in Mommy's tummy and they were always asking me how the babies were. When they found out that there wouldn't be any babies, they were really upset. My eight-year-old daughter, a week after the loss, drew a picture of angels and said, "I miss you babies, up in heaven." It just goes to show that, even though they are so young, my children did understand I had a loss and it affected them as well.

My family has been very supportive, as have my friends. Everybody took the journey with me, and everybody was devastated for me, not only with the loss, but for how I was treated and the whole situation.

I felt I really wasn't valued for what I was doing or even valued as a human being. I felt like 'hired help' and when things didn't go right, well, we'll just throw her to the curb.

If someone came to me asking whether they should be a surrogate, I would give them the opinion not to do it, but if they did, I would advise them to really think about how they could handle it if things go bad, physically and emotionally, and to protect yourself with the contract as well. The agency says you get your own lawyer, but then they appoint that lawyer for you, so that lawyer knows what they want to say. I didn't feel like I was fairly represented by someone looking out for me.

I now understand the views of those who object that surrogacy is a business transaction in which women are not treated fairly, and that laws can't protect women's health. When I delivered the babies I actually hemorrhaged and had to get an injection to stop the bleeding, but it did not stop. I lost a substantial amount of blood and had to get a blood transfusion before I left the hospital.

If I ever had the chance to talk to the intended parents, I would tell them how hurt and disappointed I am. For people that wanted a baby so badly, they were so quick just to dispose of these two 'imperfect' ones. But babies aren't disposable, they're humans and I was the one who felt life inside me. I'm the one that held the babies in my hands after I delivered them. They didn't realize what this did to me. I just don't think they deserve to be parents.

I want to get my story out into the public arena to warn people what can go wrong and to educate women who are seeking to be surrogates or who are surrogates already to protect themselves. They need to keep in mind that not all people are good and not all people have the best intentions. You just have to be really careful.

At the start, I wanted to do something great. It didn't turn out so well. You know, I was proud to be a surrogate. When I discovered the bad, it wasn't what I thought it would be, I didn't feel good about doing it anymore. I know there are still people out there who are going to say that surrogacy is a great thing, and they had a great experience. But things can go wrong and you also have to think about the egg donation side. What would that egg donor think about what happened with her genes? It's great to donate your eggs to help a woman, but then you have to think, "What is she doing with them?"

Once I decided to be a surrogate, I looked up surrogacy groups on Facebook. You don't really see anything bad out there, it's all happy stories and people supporting people. If anyone ever made one little negative comment on the Facebook group, everyone would gang up on them. I didn't go on those Facebook sites any more after my loss and I didn't say what had happened to me. I was too broken at that point. I didn't need any negative comments and I was going through so much, so I just deleted everything.

To anyone out there thinking of doing surrogacy, I would just say, you think it's going to be a happy ending, but when things go wrong, you are the one left with the effects forever. This loss is going to stay with me forever. For the intended parents, this loss is far away and it's not real. It's sad.

P.S. I need to have ongoing medical and therapy care. I have been seeing a psychiatrist and have required antidepressants and anti-anxiety medication due to depression and anxiety attacks after the loss. I have had to go on birth control to regulate my hormones due to the stress the loss put on my body and the irregular bleeding after the loss.

No Right to Know
Natascha (Russia)

As told to Eva Maria Bachinger[2]

Those of us who are surrogate mothers in Russia mostly come from country regions, or from Belarus or Ukraine. We find advertisements on the internet or in newspapers and then contact the agencies. Many of us are single mothers and we are separated from our children for many months during the pregnancy and birth of the child that we carry for the commissioning parents. At home I just said I have to go to Moscow for four months. For work. Only my mother knew the real reason. I am 30 years old and I live with my small daughter about 1000 kms from Moscow. It's a beautiful place, very green, only about 500,000 inhabitants. It takes me 30 hours by train to travel to Moscow.

During the pregnancy I lived with another surrogate mother in a flat, which the agency rented. We were not allowed to talk to each other about the details of our contracts. They are standard contracts, but they vary in details as we have to respect the wishes of the commissioning parents. So they can be quite different; expenses, abortion, yes or no. So that there is no ill will, jealousy or stuff, we are told we should not talk about the contracts. The agency offers package deals for the intended parents with a 100% baby guarantee. They can use as many egg donors or different surrogate mothers as needed until they have a baby. No extra payments required.

---

2   I conducted this interview for my 2015 book *Kind auf Bestellung. Ein Plädoyer für klare Grenzen* [Child to Order: A Plea for Clear Boundaries], Deutike Verlag, Vienna. Translation by Renate Klein.

I am not allowed to talk about where the baby was born and under what circumstances. But it was in a European capital city so that the transport over the border into the child's new country would be easy. I can't say anything about the nature of the birth or about what happens if the child has a disability. If anything is wrong the couple or the doctor decide whether an abortion is in order. I have no say in the matter. Before the surrogacy I was working as a waitress. I earned around 10,000 to 15,000 rubles a month (about 150 euros); the average income in my town is 20,000 rubles. You can survive on that sort of money. But you can't buy anything extra.

I did not select the couple. The Agency looks after people from around the world. When I was accepted by the Agency I knew nothing about the couple including where they came from. It was only when they wanted to get to know me that I found out that they came from a European country. Yes, I was very worried whether I would be able to give the child away after the birth. But then I understood that it is not my child. My egg cells are not in it. I am only a helper. So I was prepared. I knew I had to give the baby away. I knew who its parents would be and that it was expected. That made it easier. I only met the intended parents shortly before giving birth. I admit I was worried about the baby's future, but when I saw the child in the arms of the happy parents, my doubts vanished. Yes, I am in contact with them, that's how the contract stipulates it. If they want to have more contact, that's fine by me. If not, I understand. I can't answer if I want to have contact with the child one day. I don't know how I would explain to my daughter who this child is. Maybe later, when they are both grown-ups. At the moment she has no idea. When she saw me having a Skype call with the commissioning parents, I told her that it was just someone I knew. I told her I had to work in Moscow to earn more money.

I can't talk about how much money I received. It's a secret. The child I carried for the European couple is now two years and two months old. They send photographs and if they want, we talk. But the communication is irregular. It is not so easy because I only speak

Russian. I don't have any problems if the child contacts me later. I have photos that I will keep.

I have also donated egg cells but I don't know if there ever was a child. I would be pleased if it had worked. I'm not sure if I'm okay about not knowing what happened. But I guess I don't have a right to know. With the money from the surrogacy I bought myself a car. A small one, a Russian brand. I don't know if I will be a surrogate for a second time. I don't have any plans at the moment.

Bitter Family Ties:
Will I Ever See My Son Again?
Odette (Australia)

The most important thing to me, when I agreed to be a 'surrogate mother', was to be able to keep contact with my birth son and be a part of his life. But now I don't know if I will ever see my son Mitchell again, let alone hold him or touch him.

When I agreed to become a surrogate for my cousin Melanie, I was a fulltime mum living with my son Christopher, then 2 years old. My ex-partner Gary, my current partner John, my parents and John's mother were all living nearby.

Melanie and I were distant cousins, and had known each other since I was a teenager. We had remained close ever since. I looked up to her, almost like an older sister as she is 11 years older than me, and we saw each other regularly at family functions. I really loved her. I attended her wedding to Edward in 2002.

When I became pregnant with Christopher in 2012, my then partner Gary and I went to visit Melanie and Edward to share the great news in person. Ringing Melanie on our way there, she verbally abused me, was really rude and hung up on me. We were shocked at her behaviour but made excuses because we knew Melanie and her husband had been trying to have a baby without success.

Melanie did not get back in touch with me until four months later, in October 2012, to tell me she had breast cancer. She asked my opinion as to whether she should try and have embryos frozen prior to surgery and chemotherapy. She said she and Edward were happy without children but I encouraged her to have embryos frozen so that if she changed her mind later on, she could try and get pregnant then.

In mid-January 2013, I was rushed to hospital due to excessive bleeding because I suffered from placental abruption. My son Christopher was born by emergency caesarean the next day and I needed two blood transfusions to replace the lost fluids. It was a really traumatic experience but luckily Christopher was healthy. Gary and I asked Melanie and Edward to be Christopher's guardians, and they accepted.

The next few months were spent settling into our lives as parents. But in July 2014, when Christopher was 18 months old, Gary and I separated. Luckily, it was all done on good terms, and to this day we continue to share parenting responsibilities and decision-making about our son, as well as enjoying lots of activities together as a family.

In October 2014, Christopher and I were having dinner at Melanie and Edward's house when Edward said he wanted to talk to me. He explained that further IVF was out of the question for Melanie because of her cancer. He said that he and Melanie had one frozen embryo that would only be viable for at most another two years. He asked me if I would be a surrogate for them using this one embryo.

He explained that they both loved my hands-on parenting, my healthy lifestyle and diet, and my ability to teach Christopher right from wrong. They thought I was a perfect match as a surrogate for them. He even offered to pay a deposit to enable me to buy a house if I would do this for them.

I was really happy to do this, although I refused the offer of money for a house, as I just wanted to help them. I was, however, reassured that I would get the emotional and physical support I would need. They lived really close by and promised that they would visit me regularly and come to all the medical appointments. I was excited to be asked to carry a baby for them, and thought the baby would be a lovely cousin for my son. Knowing that I would always be connected to the baby, and play an active part in the child's life, was the only reason I agreed to be a surrogate.

Our first appointment with a doctor at the fertility clinic was in mid-December 2014. After initial blood tests and a physical exam, the doctor told us we needed to seek individual legal advice to draw up a surrogacy agreement. We also needed a counsellor's report. The next day, Melanie set up a bank account to enable me to access money to cover my expenses. Melanie also made an appointment for me to see a law firm, which took place in early January. Melanie and Edward's lawyers drew up a surrogacy agreement in February. They both signed it straight away.

A group counselling session, with all three of us, took place on 25 March, also organised by Melanie. This was the first counselling any of us had had. That same day, I signed the surrogacy agreement already signed a month earlier by Melanie and Edward. From that single counselling session, Mia the counsellor provided a very brief letter saying that she had no concerns about the three of us entering into a surrogacy agreement.

However, at our next appointment at the fertility clinic, the doctor expressed reservations about the qualifications of the counsellor and her extremely brief letter, aka 'report', that gave our agreement the go-ahead. Under the law, the counsellor must be accredited and Mia was not. Despite Melanie insisting the clinic accept the report, they did not, so in May we all met with an accredited counsellor who spoke to us as a group but also individually, over three hours. She submitted her report from the short session to the fertility clinic, which neither Melanie nor I saw. It was only when I requested the report, four months into my pregnancy, that I found out the second counsellor had recommended more counselling take place prior to the embryo transfer. However, this recommendation was ignored by the fertility specialist in charge. After this report was given to the fertility clinic, it was decided to go ahead with the embryo transfer scheduled for August.

In July, as part of the preparation for the transfer, I went to the clinic to commence the medication regime. The medication was never explained in detail, nor the side effects or the high dosages. I never questioned the medication as I trusted that I was being properly cared for.

The embryo transfer took place on 3 August. Melanie came with me and she was really anxious. I was positive and kept reassuring her that everything would be all right. In the days following the transfer, I was stunned that I didn't hear from either Melanie or Edward. I began to feel like I wasn't a priority for them. By the time they got in touch ten days later, I felt like I had been neglected.

My next visit to the clinic was on 18 August. My mum and my son came with me as neither Melanie nor Edward made the time. I explained to the doctor the bad side effects I was experiencing from the high levels of progesterone, including nausea, vomiting and headaches. I had done my research, and knew that the dosage was really high, compared to dosages given at other clinics in Australia and New Zealand. But the doctor totally ignored me, refusing to consider reassessing the medication. Being in his care made me very uncomfortable. I think I was treated as an infertile woman despite my natural fertility being high.

On my way back home from the clinic, I received a phone call to tell me I was four weeks pregnant. I bought flowers and a card to deliver the news to Melanie in person with my mum and son. I told her the great news and gave her a hug, but was devastated when she said, "I don't have time for this today."

On my own initiative, I changed to another fertility clinic as I couldn't cope with the medication side effects. The doctors at this second clinic viewed my side effects more seriously, including the blood spotting that was happening. During that first trimester, Melanie rang me three times to tell me that the baby was dying and I was having a miscarriage. Despite my assurances, as confirmed by medical tests that the baby was fine, she refused to believe them. She disagreed with my decision to change clinics too. I had had a miscarriage once before due to domestic violence, so I was really upset about all these calls from her. A woman who had never been able to conceive a child at all, was cold-heartedly telling me that I was miscarrying. There were no thoughts or care given to my emotions or health at the time.

At the first ultrasound, Melanie refused to take the photo offered to us, saying that the baby would die anyway. Edward later confided in me that he was concerned about how negative Melanie was feeling about my pregnancy and that she wasn't able to handle the fact that I could carry their child and she could not. He also said he didn't really want a baby at all and it had all been Melanie's idea. All of this made me angry and distressed.

Things only got worse as the pregnancy progressed. Edward became annoyed at having to take time off work to attend appointments, so I began to attend many of them on my own. When later in the year I purchased a house with my de facto John, they refused to help us move, even though just a few months previously, they had offered me money for a house deposit. I didn't understand these changed attitudes at all but they were hurtful. Then we found out I was having a boy. Melanie was really disappointed and said she had wanted a girl. It made me really upset that she was acting in such a selfish and entitled way.

I never thought before getting pregnant that Melanie would abandon me and the unborn baby. But as soon as the embryo transfer happened she started to distance herself from us. At first I did not understand why because I thought they wanted a child. Now I feel that Melanie asked me to carry a baby, but then harboured resentment towards me for doing what she had asked me because she couldn't be pregnant. I was on the receiving end of verbal and mental abuse throughout my entire pregnancy.

We attended some more counselling sessions with Mia (whom we all liked despite the fact she wasn't properly accredited) and I confided in her privately that Melanie's treatment of me made me regret the surrogacy arrangement. This then became a point of contention when Mia told Melanie what I had said. It resulted in a shouting match on the phone, with Melanie being very abusive. I realised then that not once had Melanie ever said 'thank you' to me for doing this surrogacy for her. With the stress of our relationship, and my extreme sickness such as vomiting which was continuing, I rang the clinic in the aftermath of the phone call to inquire about an abortion. They told me we could discuss it at our next appointment. I never followed up on this request, as it was made on the spur of the moment after the terrible phone call with Melanie. It was a passing thought that I never acted on. However, I did feel really trapped, given the now toxic relationship between Melanie, Edward and I. The obstetrician spoke sternly to Edward about the need to protect me, and the baby, from Melanie's bad behaviour. She explained that high stress during the pregnancy was harmful to the unborn child which could lead to lifelong problems. I wondered how we would ever sort it out.

In mid-December, Melanie reached out to me asking if she and Edward could visit. Even though I hadn't seen Melanie since I was 12 weeks pregnant, I agreed, thinking that Melanie must have gotten help for her mental problems and that she was going to enjoy the rest of the journey with me. On the day that was arranged by Melanie, only Edward arrived. I asked him where Melanie was and he told me that she had a headache. Meanwhile, here I was still constantly nauseous, with headaches and vomiting. I was growing a baby, looking after my three-year-old son by myself and running a household. I sent a package of baby gifts back with Edward to give to Melanie. I did not receive any acknowledgement or thanks. I was really disappointed, as things obviously weren't improving between us. Edward told me Melanie had decided to keep away from me as it was too hard on her me being pregnant.

A couple of days later, I received an email from the Attorney-General's Department saying that Melanie had contacted them asking them to resolve a dispute between us. This caused me great distress, considering Edward had been in my house two days prior and not mentioned a word of this. I could not get a lawyer's appointment until late January given it was the Christmas holiday period. In the meantime, Melanie drained the bank account she had set up for me, meaning that I had to meet many costs myself, everything from petrol to medical tests. I had already paid for things before, but now finances were becoming really difficult, with new out-of-pocket expenses. Then my lawyers told me that Melanie and Edward would no longer pay any of my legal fees, despite them having agreed to do so. I began to really worry where things were heading so I contacted Adoptions Services, Queensland, to discuss the option of an open adoption if the surrogacy arrangement fell through.

Just two days prior to my 28-week scan I had an unexpected phone call from Melanie. She was shouting down the line stating I had been nothing but rude to her during the pregnancy. I tried to explain to her that her constant negative attitude and telling me the baby I was carrying would die, was extremely upsetting and stressful for me and the baby. I listened to her tirade on speaker phone so my partner John heard everything. However, I decided I would extend one last olive branch and offered for Melanie and Edward to attend the upcoming scan. On the day, Edward entered the clinic alone. I asked him where Melanie was and he told me she was waiting outside. When the obstetrician called us into the appointment Edward went outside to get Melanie. She entered the room and refused to acknowledge me. In response, the doctor asked them to leave as she didn't think it was beneficial for my, or the baby's health, to have them present for the rest of the consultation. With the doctor, I discussed the birth plan, which included her advice to have a Caesarean. Melanie was furious about not being involved in these discussions. She and Edward tried to interfere with my birthing plans, bombarding the hospital with emails, as well as logging on using my details to change my post-birth accommodation arrangements to a smaller apartment. I instructed the hospital not to divulge further details to them. Having Melanie use my personal details to gain information made me feel quite threatened.

In February, through my lawyer, I wrote Melanie and Edward a letter informing them that I wanted no further contact with them until the baby was born. Correspondence about mediation went back and forth between our lawyers, but their lawyers determined that mediation before the birth of the baby would be unhelpful.

By March, my out-of-pocket expenses were around $4000 and mounting. More correspondence between our lawyers followed. Via them I was told that any expenses would only be paid once the baby was handed over into the care of Melanie and Edward, and once I had signed a parentage order. If I didn't hand over the baby or consent to a parentage order, we would be 'in litigation mode.' This came just one week before the baby was due and being threatened with legal action really upset me.

I was still considering the adoption option, and I was visited by Adoption Services, Queensland to discuss it further. The most important issue for me was to keep contact with the baby. I was told I would have a big part in the selection of his parents if I went ahead with the adoption.

My baby boy was born via planned Caesarean on 11 April 2016 at 2pm, weighing a healthy 7 pound 9 ounces. I received flowers from Edward and Melanie, to me a thoughtless gift to save face. I asked mum to take the flowers back to Melanie and to request her to pay the expenses. But I consented to the baby staying overnight with Edward and Melanie in the hospital.

The day after the birth, I was unable to move because of the surgery, and I asked for the baby to be returned to my room. He came to me with hardly any clothes on – Melanie had refused to clothe the baby as she didn't want me having the clothes – and with terrible wind.

I noticed on my birth son's chart that he had been given one bottle of milk formula for the first 24 hours and then was changed to another brand. When I questioned the midwife about this, she informed me that Melanie hadn't been prepared for his arrival and that she had only brought in formula that afternoon. I found this particularly upsetting as Melanie told me when I was 12 weeks pregnant that I would give birth to a stillborn baby, and she would not be getting anything prepared for the baby's arrival. There had been several legal letters requesting confirmation that Melanie and Edward were ready – and we had been told they were. However, the evidence proved that they were not ready for the baby at all.

My birth son spent the second night with me but I learnt from hospital staff the next day that Melanie had called the police citing fears for the baby's safety while in my care. My lawyer emailed requesting urgent mediation. That same day, a woman tried to subpoena me while I was in my hospital bed. My lawyer accepted it on my behalf. I learnt that accusations of child abuse were now being levelled at me. I was devastated to learn of such heinous false allegations. Where did they even come from?

Nevertheless, my son stayed with me for the next two nights. The court mediation hearing was set for 11am on 14th April. For me, it took place over the phone as I was still in hospital. I had to make a decision as to whether I should fight for the rights of the baby I had nurtured and carried for nine months, or put my first son and family first. John had suggested we keep the baby and raise him as our own, but I knew we couldn't afford to fight the case in court. Plus I thought a fresh start in a new family via adoption might be best for my birth son, without all the negativity and tension that had surrounded the pregnancy.

On 15th April, the Family Court made interim orders to allow Melanie and Edward to make an application for a parentage order, which is allowed under the Queensland Surrogacy Act 2010. This had been agreed upon during a mediation session on the 14th April. Melanie and Edward requested that the baby be called Mitchell, with no middle name, and stated that he would carry my surname, which was the correct thing to do as I was listed as his birth mother on the birth certificate. When Mitchell was collected on 15 April by a nurse to be given to Melanie and Edward, I didn't agree with him going to them, as I didn't think it was in his best interests. But I had to put the needs of Christopher first and I was not able to afford the tens of thousands of dollars it would have cost to fight in the family court to keep Mitchell safe with Christopher, John and I. All the baby things I had given to them to help care for Mitchell were returned to me except for clothing, along with a note from Melanie which said, "I will tell our child how wonderful you are and I am sure when he is older he would love to meet you." So much for the prospect of playing a big part in Mitchell's life, as I had been led to expect.

Post-birth, I was unable to drive for six weeks and bled for 12, while taking three courses of antibiotics for internal infections and haemorraghing. I also sported a new Caesarian scar, as they did not cut in the same place as when Christopher was delivered. But it was Mitchell's health that worried me most. I have not been able to see him or hold him or touch him since he was taken from me that day in hospital, 15th April 2016. My trauma was compounded by a scare four months after I gave birth that I may have ovarian cancer; a cancer which might be caused by some of the medications I had received during the pregnancy. I continued to bleed for more than a year right up until July 2017. Since the birth, I have undergone four ultrasounds and two Pap smear tests trying to find out what had gone wrong.

Melanie and Edward paid some of my invoices that I sent to them although it was far short of what I was owed. But they gave no news of Mitchell and did not acknowledge my emails inquiring after his health, how he was growing and whether he had received his immunisations. I asked for a photo but never got one. I received a Mother's Day card in 2016 from them but Mitchell's name was conspicuously omitted from it. I felt the card gesture was totally insincere.

In July, via my lawyer, I learnt that they requested I not contact them at all. I was really upset as all I wanted was to learn how my baby was going and I was being totally ignored. In one email I sent them in August, I asked, "How is baby Mitchell going? Is he crawling? I am concerned for his welfare and want to know how he is going. Would be nice if you let me know. He would be gaining weight nicely since I gave birth to him. Give him a cuddle from his Tummy Mummy and let him know we love him." This email was never acknowledged and I was now becoming distraught.

Then I learned that they had changed Mitchell's name to Kieran, contrary to the court order and what was on his birth certificate. And despite them specifically requesting I name him for them. I imagined my birth son's confusion and that really worried me. But this was just one hurdle in the nightmare of legal proceedings that then followed.

Via lawyers, a counsellor was engaged to write a mandatory report under the Queensland Surrogacy Act 2010 for the purposes of obtaining a parentage order. Ms West met with Melanie and Edward in August 2016, and with me in September 2016. The purpose of a parentage order would be to transfer parentage from me to Edward and Melanie. It would also mean that a new birth certificate would be issued for Mitchell aka Kieran with their names on it. I was forced to meet with Ms West by my lawyer who said that if I didn't meet with her I would be seen as uncooperative, and Melanie and Edward would have no choice but to proceed with the Family Court, even though their lawyers were threatening to forgo the Parentage Order and proceed to the Family Court anyway. This is despite the fact that I was still thousands of dollars in debt from unpaid expenses due to ongoing medical issues from the birth and, of course, mounting legal costs. Ms West was quite unaware of the threats coming from Melanie's legal team and she had no idea of the name change from Mitchell to Kieran. Melanie and Edward had lied to her during their face-to-face encounter.

Ms West's report, which was submitted to the Family Court by a sworn affidavit in December 2016, reflected this. It also contained the false claims of Melanie and Edward that they had paid for an overseas holiday for my family. If they had paid for it, this would have amounted to a 'Commercial Surrogacy', which is a criminal offence in all of Australia and in Queensland under the Surrogacy Act 2010. I could not believe the lies that were being told and I provided evidence to my lawyer showing that the holiday had been paid from John's wages.

When our extended family learned about the court proceedings, some offered to pay the money that Melanie and Edward owed me. Although they thought that they were solving the problem, I found it rather insulting. Melanie has always been fortunate in life and even now, with her deciding not to pay her debts, she had others offering to pay them for her. I refused their offer.

The next months were punctuated by phone calls and letters between lawyers, counsellors and medicos. Despite my attempts, via phone and email, to receive news about Mitchell and to get my expenses paid, I did not hear from either Edward or Melanie. The lack of any information about Mitchell really weighed heavily on my mind and I worried about the level of care he was receiving. I learnt that, instead of communicating with me, they were going to proceed straight to the Family Court to litigate the surrogacy arrangement. They thought they would be able to obtain an order removing my human rights as a birth mother.

I had always wanted to be part of Mitchell's life and to have him as part of my family with Christopher. I needed Mitchell to know that I had not abandoned him; that I love him and care for him. I registered with Children's Contact Services in an effort to gain assistance to have contact with my baby. But if the Family Court ruled in favour of Melanie and Edward, I faced the prospect that the undertakings that had been given to me from the start about being involved in the baby's life, may well be overruled. I felt I was being blackmailed into signing the parentage order to avoid the Family Court proceedings – but I could not sign the order while I had no news of the baby and the expenses were left unpaid. Yet the prospect of fighting it out in court terrified me. There was no right answer. Then Melanie laid a complaint against my lawyer and with unpaid bills for legal fees now totalling $12,000, my lawyer told me he could no longer represent me. I felt totally abandoned. By October 2016, I was on anxiety medication prescribed by my GP. I still had no news about the baby and emailed Melanie and Edward again. All I received was an email from their lawyers asking me not to contact them further.

Not being able to see my birth son Mitchell or know how he is doing was very traumatizing for me. Christopher and I had spent many months talking to him regularly during the pregnancy and bonding with him. I remained his legal mother with the court case pending – yet I didn't even have a photo of him. A couple of months after the hospital ordeal, a nurse approached me to inform me of an incident that had occurred while Mitchell was in the care of Melanie and Edward on the first night after his birth. This led to staff calling child services and filing a report (which came to nothing as the director backtracked, but the nurse's concerns were backed up later in court documents). The concern was that Melanie had refused to cuddle Mitchell with skin to skin contact. When Mitchell did not stop screaming, Edward jumped up on the couch, ripped his shirt open and yelled "I will do it then." When I heard this, it triggered an anxiety attack. I was – and remain – so fearful of my son not being loved. (And this wasn't the only complaint filed by nursing staff against Melanie.)

Around this time I learnt that the Family Court would need accurate evidence of Mitchell's biological parentage as part of the case. Reflecting on the period when I had become pregnant, I realised I had had sex with John at the time of conception and it dawned on me for the first time that perhaps Mitchell was not the biological son of Melanie and Edward at all. The potential impacts were huge. This led to more legal complications, as our various lawyers debated the merits of DNA testing for all of us, plus who would meet the expenses of all these tests. The uncertainty about the baby's genetic origins added to my hardship and made it almost impossible to provide instructions to my lawyers about my preferred course of action in the upcoming court case. Until the test results were known in February, it was as if we were all collectively holding our breath. When they came through, Melanie and Edward were confirmed as the baby's genetic parents. But I still wanted to be part of Mitchell's life. It was me that had grown him from my own blood and bones; I was his birth mother. It was now approaching a year since his birth and I had not seen him – or a picture – since he was taken from me in the hospital.

Our case was heard in the Family Court in February 2017, after the DNA results were known, but the judgment was not handed down until September 2017. It was devastating news. Edward and Melanie were given sole parenting responsibility for baby Mitchell. However, the irony was that I remained as my son's birth mother on the birth certificate. Yet I was not allowed to see him unless Melanie and Edward agreed. His name on the birth certificate would be changed to Kieran, not Mitchell or Junior or other names he had been called. They had already changed his name despite the earlier court order from April 14 2016. I was given no rights whatsoever to care for, access, visit or even see photos of my son. In fact, because I had been denied any access to Mitchell after his birth, this was then used against me in the court case. As the court could not establish an ongoing relationship between us – because I had been denied the contact I was promised – this then strengthened Edward and Melanie's case in wanting to be fully and solely responsible for him. The fact that he had spent three nights with me after the birth counted for nothing. During the hearing we also discovered that Melanie had threatened both her life and mine more than once which resulted in her being admitted to the local hospital's mental health ward. This was troubling to find out: that this woman who we heard was rocking herself on the floor in numerous mental breakdowns was now the sole carer for Mitchell/Kieran. Plus she had access to fire-arms kept in their home!

Bizarrely, the judge also ruled that Mitchell/Kieran not having any contact with me, his birth mother, would not have any impact on his life at all. But having me on his birth certificate was okay. Knowing that one day he will find out about me and be told utter lies is harrowing. I hope he doesn't feel I abandoned him.

Because of the surrogacy and ongoing stress and trauma after my baby was born, John and I have split up, which perhaps is not so surprising. I am so sad about what has happened with this surrogacy – but also angry. I feel betrayed, hurt, and I am still suffering mentally and physically from what I have been through. I have great trouble sleeping. Not a day goes by that I do not regret handing over Mitchell in the hospital. I regret not fighting for him after his birth. Not a day goes by where I do not think about him and wonder if he is safe.

I understand from reading the laws and regulations about surrogacy that protecting the rights of the child should be paramount. I also understand that 'birth mothers' like me should not be exploited. But that is exactly what I feel has happened.

I have also learnt that a baby develops better by having an ongoing relationship with his or her birth mother. I know from other surrogates' experiences that their birth children never forget their birth mothers and that the bond they hold is for life. It is also cited in many laws concerning children that they should have an ongoing relationship with their birth parent(s). It also clearly states in the law that the child should have an ongoing relationship with the surrogate whenever possible.

After the devastating judgment in September 2017, I was trying to process what had happened. The only good thing was that I found a wonderful new lawyer who continued to fight for me. And she does it all pro bono because she passionately believes that great injustice has been done to my birth son and me. The next step was to appeal the Family Court Judge's verdict.

In January 2018, we appeared before the Full Bench of the Family Court of Australia for the appeal on the legal basis that the judge in the trial allowed Edward to be put on the birth certificate as the father even though, in our reading of the law, he is only considered a sperm donor.

During the hearing, the barrister for Melanie and Edward requested that I pay both their existing legal costs and future legal costs, or if the judge was found to have erred in his judgment, then they wanted the Commonwealth to pay costs. This was requested even after my barrister had informed the judge that I was a single mother on the pension, and she was working on a pro bono basis. This information had been conveyed to the other barrister before the hearing but was ignored and they sought costs from me regardless.

The Court of Appeal came back with a verdict in March 2018, saying that the judge had erred in his decision. Our case was set for a re-trial. The issue of costs was also discussed, with the judges acknowledging that legal costs rested with Melanie and Edward, stating:

> In the result the appeal has succeeded, but on a point not raised in the written submissions of the parties and not raised below. In any event, the appellant was represented pro bono and costs were not sought if the appeal succeeded.
>
> Although costs certificates were sought for the appeal and the rehearing, it is not appropriate that public funds be expended in circumstances where the proceedings have miscarried as a result of the parties' failure to address the relevant statutory requirements.

In May 2018 we had a hearing with the original judge for a time-line of all legal arguments to be submitted. My barrister submitted a strong legal argument discussing the Queensland Surrogacy Act 2010 and the Status of Children's Act 1978, arguing that Edward cannot be both a parent and an intending parent of the child. However, Melanie and Edward's barrister submitted that John was not the birth father, the legal costs were unfair (pointing out again that my barrister was working pro bono), and argued that I was undertaking this legal action purely out of anger.

Yet in Queensland, all lawyers are entitled to act on a pro bono case, especially when there are special circumstances. Given that my case was a first under Queensland law, this assistance to me was totally appropriate.

Melanie's and Edward's lawyers also argued that it would be in Mitchell/Kieran's best interests to have one of his biological parents on his birth certificate, maintaining that since his certificate carried 'only' my name, this would be confusing for him later in life. What they seemed to have forgotten is that there is a multitude of evidence in the international literature that denying a child a relationship with their birth mother can result in long-term mental and emotional suffering. I think the best interests of Mitchell/Kieran have been ignored from the start.

In August 2018, the judge delivered his judgment in writing. He rejected all our arguments and re-issued his original order that the sperm donor, Edward, was to be entered as Mitchell/Kieran's father on the child's birth certificate. Because the various laws in Queensland are indeed contradictory, his rationale for doing so relied on his belief that Edward being called Mitchell's 'father' on the birth certificate was in the child's best interest. He also stated that he believed the appeal should not have been successful.

His initial order that I was to have no contact with my birth son unless approved by Melanie and Edward, still stands. I am left as the birthmother on the birth certificate. A mother without the right to even see a photo of her birth son, let alone see and cuddle him. What a sad joke.

This is the end of the legal road for us although my lawyer has vowed to approach the Queensland Attorney General about the injustice of it all.

I am still left with $20,000 of unpaid medical and legal bills. But much worse, I am left with deep regret and a neverending sadness at the prospect of not seeing my birth son until he is 18, when he might access his birth certificate and find my name listed as his birth mother.

I have moved as I am fearful of my family's security; I felt it was the only option. My cousin is still determined to ruin my life. She has set up social media accounts using my name to further inflict pain on me and my friends. By doing this she is committing a criminal offence and I was in the process of filing criminal charges. But then I felt that this may impact both Christopher's and my safety. At least it is all recorded with the police.

My heart is broken, knowing that I won't get any news from Mitchell, not even a picture of what he looks like. I will continue to send things to him. They might not reach him, but Melanie and Edward can never say I did not try.

When I hear people say "Oh, there is nothing wrong with altruistic surrogacy, it's commercial surrogacy that is more problematic," I want to scream. I am not the only birth mother in Australia who embarked on a family surrogacy because we wanted to help relatives who could not have children. I did it out of love and thinking my first son would be able to grow up with a special cousin. My genuine offer to help has been repaid with unbelievable cruelty that will be with me for the rest of my life. I have been forced to abandon my birth son.

Would I suggest to any woman she should become a surrogate out of love? Not anymore. My story shows that it is wrong to ask a woman to grow a baby for nine months, give birth to the child and then face the possibility of not having any news or seeing them for years to come. As women we deserve better, we are not just baby carriers but human beings with a lot of love to give.

Sadly, I feel I will never recover from this nightmare. Every day I think about my son, the son I can't see or touch. Christopher also suffers from not knowing and asks where is the baby and why can't we see him? I am very open about what has happened and explain it to Christopher – just without names. The second scar on my body is another daily reminder of what I have lost. Not to mention the anxiety and depression that I now suffer from these traumatic experiences. The surrogacy has torn our once close family apart. Nobody talks about this so-called miracle or asks why I am not in Mitchell/Kieran's life. It's our family's dirty secret. I worry about what my son will think when he discovers the truth and what lies he will be told. Forever in my heart dear Mitchell, so much love for you my son.

When My Surrogacy Became My Nightmare
Denise (USA)

My husband heard about surrogacy from a customer where he worked. We thought this was a great way for us to help our family and help another family at the same time and made the decision to move forward.

I became a surrogate in 2016 for a couple in China and initially everything went well. I had two transfers, the first failed but the second one was a success. And at six weeks they saw a second heart beat, and told me that "one embryo had split into two identical twins."

However, it was very clear on the ultrasound that the embryos were in two separate sacs. So it was strange that I was told they were identical when they were in two sacs. My pregnancy went well but I had to contemplate my first ever surgery at 30 years old, a C-section. I was told as it was twins, I could not push them out.

On 12 December 2016, I went in for a scheduled C-section at 38 weeks pregnant. Afterwards, I did not see the babies as they were immediately rolled away with their new 'mom'. When I was taken to my room after recovery the intended mother and my caseworker came in to say hi. I asked her if I could see a picture of the babies, and the mother handed me her phone. I looked at the babies, then handed her phone back and said, "They look different!"

The intended mother said nothing, but my caseworker stated that she too had carried identical twins that came out looking very different but became identical as they got older ... Two days passed by and the intended mother Yu Yan (a pseudonym) checked in on me twice a day and each time I asked to see pictures and she seemed to become very bothered by it. One time she handed me her phone and said, "Are you satisfied now?"

I was in a lot of pain and on pain medication and very tired, so I didn't think anything of it. On her last visit, I asked her if she was going to bring the babies by so I could say goodbye to them? She stated "probably not" and that hurt me deeply. I immediately fell into a big depression because I just sacrificed my health and nine months of my life to bless her with having a family and she couldn't even give me the pleasure to kiss these babies goodbye and wish them good luck.

Later, I realized that in my contract, it says that I am to have a one-hour visit with the babies before leaving the hospital. The intended mother did not abide by that nor did my case worker make sure that everything was being done as stated in my contract.

A month went by and Yu Yan finally sent me some pictures of both of the babies. She asked me if anything looks different to me? I said yes, they look different, as I had already stated in the hospital! She said that she had been waiting for me to feel better before she wanted to let me know that she is having doubts that one baby clearly isn't Chinese and believes it isn't hers. She told me they were waiting for the DNA results before their embassy would let them take the babies home.

By this time I am freaking out! About a week later, I get a picture of the DNA results that the Chinese intended father is not the genetic father of one baby. I immediately called my caseworker to find out what the hell is going on and how can this be! She couldn't answer anything! My caseworker immediately goes and picks up the baby and takes him under her care since it was clear this baby did not belong to this Chinese family. The caseworker then made an appointment for me and the baby to get tested.

I made it to my appointment but my caseworker did not make it to the baby's appointment. So, here I am, still stuck in shock and wonder and finally after days of waiting, I got the results that I *am* the genetic mother of this baby! And DNA testing proved my husband is the genetic father!

In disbelief and heartbreak, I do not know what to do. My caseworker tried to talk my husband and me into allowing them to give my boy up for adoption, because, she says, whoever takes him will be responsible for paying back over $20,000 to the Chinese couple as they say they didn't want to have to pay for me to deliver my own baby. The caseworker also told me that she wants me to reimburse her for caring for my son since she had to pay out of her own pocket for food, diapers, clothes and a baby car seat.

Now, we are a middle class family, who did not have a dime to pay back and we had just bought a house a couple of weeks before this happened. The surrogate agency tried to work the process out without legal representation, which was another breach of my contract. They wanted me to sign an agreement before they gave me my own child!

I made call after call, but no one knew what to do because they had never heard of my kind of story before. It is a rare occurrence called *superfetation*, where a woman while already pregnant, can get pregnant again! The agency was accusing me of not abiding by the terms of my contract, to not have sexual intercourse with my husband until a positive pregnancy test confirmed that I was pregnant. But I swear, I fully kept to all the terms in my contract. I must already have been pregnant before the embryo transfer.

We finally found an attorney who would take on my case. After reading the agreement, she stated she had never seen anything so ridiculous in her 15 years of practice. She sent the surrogacy agency an email letting them know that if they do not hand over my child, they will create more damage than they already have for themselves. So the agency finally contacted me, and told me where to meet my caseworker to get my son.

By this time, we have nothing for this poor baby, we had to make calls to friends with young children, asking them if they had anything they weren't using anymore. My own children were already six and two years old. We were supposed to get my son back several times, but they always had an excuse to prolong the process and trying to get money from us. They lied and said the intended parents wanted to adopt him out, so they can get their money back and since they had signed his birth certificate, they were his legal parents and had that right.

Another time, they told us they didn't want to sign the power of attorney. So many lies! Three weeks passed with me and my husband living with the knowledge that I carried our own child for nine and a half months and now he's almost two months old and he is still not living with us. I felt just so totally sick – emotionally and physically.

We finally got to hold our son when he was eight weeks old. Meanwhile, the surrogate agency has an attorney that is still making my life a living hell. He wrote a two-page letter to my attorney stating nothing but lies about me. He also filed a false complaint about me, that wasn't true, because he was upset that we had set up a gofundme account to raise money to pay our own attorney's fees.

Fast forward to today. Our son is now eight months old, and he is healthy, beautiful, and happy. But now we are in debt with attorney fees, although she didn't even finish the job we hired her to do.

The surrogate agency continues to blame me for getting pregnant with my own child. By now I have done my research and know that this can in fact happen to women. They should have informed me that this could occur, even if it is rare!

If the caseworker was overseeing the process as she should have been, and allowed me to see the babies immediately after their birth I would have known right away that something was wrong. This agency allowed my baby boy to be taken from the hospital by another woman, allowed her to sign his birth certificate, and give him a Chinese name and then after proof he was mine they held him ransom for three weeks!

It is inhumane and sickening what has happened to my family, my baby and me! I am truly heartbroken that this is how they repay me for what I have done to give them a child. I was a victim of child kidnapping and asking for ransom and no one helped me. I am still reaching out for help or direction to bring justice for what they have allowed to be done. They have no clue how much pain and stress they created for me. They have mentally damaged me and created a lot of pain for my family. I am a woman of God and truly believe that it is God who has given me back my baby boy.

I now have a corrected birth certificate for my child with his true name on it. But I am still devastated. If surrogacy can lead to so much trouble and pain then I think it should not be allowed.

I Am an Incubator
Natalia (Russia)
As told to Eva Maria Bachinger[3]

Natalia arrives with her husband. They live in a block of flats in a downtrodden part of Moscow. They have suggested we meet in a shopping centre. But when I get there it is deafeningly noisy. Men dressed as Spiderman and Batman shout into microphones to encourage children to play. There are no cafés here and it's rather unpleasant to contemplate a walk. The weather is cold and humid. The remaining snow has turned black. Cars speed along on the freeway; drivers don't care that they drive through potholes of brown sludge. Pedestrians have to move to the side to avoid getting wet.

The baby growing in my tummy is the child of a 36-year-old Russian woman who lives with her husband in an expensive part of Moscow. I don't know any more and I don't want to know more. No one knows about my pregnancy, only my husband. No one must know about it. I am five months' pregnant but it's hard to see a baby bump. Many people think I am younger than I am. When I put on make-up I look a bit older. My husband's and my son is ten years old. I was a very young mother but that was no problem as we already lived in the same apartment.

Obviously I eat well, I don't smoke, and I don't drink alcohol. I am a responsible person. When I have reached 36 weeks I am required to

---

3   I conducted this interview for my 2015 book *Kind auf Bestellung. Ein Plädoyer für klare Grenzen* [Child to Order: A Plea for Clear Boundaries], Deutike Verlag, Vienna. Sentences in italics are my comments. Translation by Renate Klein.

stay in Moscow. In the contract it says I have to attend lots of medical appointments but I only go to the clinic for a check-up once a month. It's handy that the clinic is around the corner from the apartment that the clinic is providing for us during the duration of the pregnancy.

As a matter of fact I wanted to donate egg cells but they would not let me. I don't know why not. Then they suggested I could work as a surrogate mother and we decided to do that. We try not to take everything too seriously and we laugh a lot. We are not really thinking a lot about what's happening – what is the point? I will get a million rubles (about 12,000 euros) after the birth, and already now 20,000 rubles a month. We want to buy a house. It's our only chance to earn so much money so fast. We would have to rob a bank because we simply will not get a loan from them. We don't have a stable income. My husband works as a casual labourer in the construction industry when there is work. I study law.

I was simply looking for a way to earn good money. We are realists, there is no other way. Because of the changing value of the ruble, we are not sure if this will be enough money for a house and we are worried. But we can always do some of the work ourselves. My husband can do anything with his hands! I've deferred my studies but in the future I would like to work as a lawyer for the police. No one is worried that we are not home because we are often away for months. We need to go to places where there is work for my husband. My son always stays with my mother.

Will the child contact me one day? That's in the realm of fantasy. The parents won't ever tell the child how it came into this world. That's why I am not thinking about it. It's private. It's a secret. That's why I don't want any contact with the intending parents, I do what they want. If they change their mind and want contact, that's not a problem for me. The surrogacy contract is very simple and quite ambiguous. If there is a problem, the contract can be interpreted in this way or that. For me the most important thing is that the contract states how much money I will be paid at the end. I am not sure what would happen if the child has a disability because there is nothing in the contract about that. I am critical of this because it leaves things very unclear. But then it's how we live our lives here: problems are discussed when and if they arise. People keep quiet and if there is a problem they say, "Oh, you didn't know that?" But prenatal tests exclude disability, and PID (preimplantation genetic diagnosis) was done before the embryo transfer. There was also sex selection. I do feel a bit different during this pregnancy because it's a girl, but otherwise it's all the same as when I was pregnant with my son.

I am not walking around thinking "I am pregnant because of the money." I am just simply pregnant. I am an incubator, the vessel for this child. The doctor told me already in the 14th week that it was a girl. She said, the baby is really small, only her lips are big and full. We are planning a natural birth. I am not thinking about how it will be when the baby is taken away immediately afterwards. I am not a sentimental person. It's important for me that the child is healthy. After that this is finished for me. I'm done. We will take the first train to get out of Moscow.

Exploited, Lied to, Financially Ruined and Devastated
Kelly (USA)[4]

My first surrogacy journey should have been a huge red flag to me. But I didn't learn. I love being pregnant, I love excitement, I love people fussing over baby bellies and I love happy endings, you know.

My first surrogacy went like this. I saw an ad in my local paper. I was living in Iowa. My brother had just committed suicide in May of 2004. The ad was from an agency out of Indianapolis. "Surrogate mothers needed," it read. I had written a report in high school on surrogacy and was against it. So many babies already exist that need homes. But after having two kids of my own and seeing people with fertility issues and the hoops to jump through to adopt, I thought what a gift I can be part of. This baby will look like them, or their egg donor. Not like me. It won't be my baby.

I called the agency. I spoke to what I then thought was a wonderful woman named Linda. She worked for an attorney who owned the agency. I was sent this huge application form to fill out and then wait to hear from them. On my application I indicated that I would not work with a gay couple. I lived in a very small community in a very Catholic town. I was not going to bring that sort of attention on myself.

Well, the agency called with a match almost immediately. A gay couple from Paris. They told me the couple was married. They gave

4   Kelly's story can be viewed in full in the 2018 film documentary *#BigFertility*, written, produced and directed by Jennifer Lahl of The Center for Bioethics and Culture. <www.cbc-network.org>

me this story of how amazing this couple was and how people would not help them because they were gay. I felt bad. I was on such a rush about all this, I talked my husband Jay into it. The agency sent me a video of the 'glorious journey' I was about to embark on. The attorney was featured in it, and I was informed that I could claim all the costs on taxes and that I could use my maternity allowance on clothes or a new couch – it didn't matter what. I was told my name would not go on the birth certificate. We went to Oregon to meet the couple and the doctors that were involved. The couple paid for everything. It was a go. I started my medications and cycle.

The night before we were due to leave, Linda called me and said something had come up and my name needed to go on the birth certificate. If I did not agree to this I would not be able to continue the journey and I would need to pay back everything the couple had already paid for – the trip to Oregon, the trip to Indianapolis, where we had visited the agency, all of it. We did not have this kind of money. I talked to Jay and we were like "I guess." So we went for the embryo transfer in Oregon at a clinic the Paris couple selected because of their success rates.

Two embryos were placed in my womb; both took the very first time. The couple was nice. I thought I would be able to extend my family. Closer to delivery, Linda called again and said that immediately after the twins were born I would need to accompany the couple to Des Moines in Iowa to get the birth certificates. I delivered the babies on 8 December. One C-section, one vaginal birth. This made my recovery a little harder. But, we did what Linda said and we went to Des Moines. Then Linda calls again. Something else 'unexpected' came up and I would need to go to Chicago now with the couple to obtain the passports for the babies or they couldn't leave the United States. Jay, my husband, was pissed. We loaded up our own two children aged three and one, with me battling an infection from the C-section and headed to Chicago: over 300 miles away which took us more than five hours. The couple called us in the hotel and wanted to meet for dinner and 'debrief' me!

We met at Denny's. This was the very first time we were informed of the 'story'.

Since surrogacy is illegal in France, we were going to go to the French Consulate and tell them that I had met Philippe (the older bald one) at a bar in Waterloo (Iowa). I was to say that I cheated on my husband and became pregnant with twins. I could not keep them if I wanted to save my marriage so I had decided to send the twins to live in Paris with their father and I would visit regularly.

You should have seen Jay's face! I was totally mortified. If we didn't do this, the twins could not go to Paris. We did not finish dinner. We headed back to the hotel room. I tried and tried to get a hold of my attorney but it was late at night. The next day we met the couple at the building that housed the French Consulate. We went in and headed towards the elevator. The couple told Jay he could not go in – only Philippe and myself. They handed me a car seat. The elevator door closed. 37th floor. We stepped off. Everything was in French. Here I was with babies, car seat and a diaper bag. The entire meeting was in French. I don't speak French, so I had no idea what was said. The Consulate lady and Philippe exchanged conversation and would look at me and laugh. I was scared to death. I never said a word. I signed some papers, all in French and shook hands and headed to the elevator. When we got down to the main floor Jay was very upset. The guys thanked us and went to shake Jay's hand and he looked right at them and said, "We are done!"

I finally got hold of my attorney and he said, "What the hell did you just do?" I terminated my parental rights in Iowa immediately. The couple said as soon as they got back to Paris they would have my name removed from the birth certificate. They never did. And I found out later that they were not legally married. They called me a couple years ago and wanted to pay for me to go to Chicago and do an adoption proceeding saying I could not be the mother anymore. I declined. To this day I don't know if these children still have my name on their birth certificates in France.

I decided to get some counseling to help me deal with all the issues of losing my mother, my father and my brother. I went to see a counselor who knew that I had been a surrogate, and she actually told me about another couple she was counseling who needed a surrogate and suggested I help them have a baby. In retrospect I think it was unethical of her to do that when I came to her for help with my grief ...

But eventually I thought that my first surrogacy was just a one-off bad experience and that this next time everything would be fine. We didn't go through an agency and used the couple's attorney to draw up the contract. The intended mother had to be hospitalized for very bad Ovarian Hyperstimulation Syndrome (OHSS) after the egg retrieval and I was worried to go through with the embryo transfer. But she insisted she would be fine and to go ahead. I did get pregnant and delivered a single baby girl. A little while after the baby was born, the couple divorced, so I have some guilt about the fact that at first the baby was so wanted and now is being raised by her father.

Money plays a big role in surrogacy. If there were no money in surrogacy I would never have done it. But money was tight for us, so I decided to be a surrogate again. This time I worked with an agency because I thought there would be protections for me in case something went wrong. The agency matched me with a heterosexual couple in Spain. We chatted on Skype; it wasn't a warm connection, more like, "let's work together." I got pregnant with twins for them. When it came time in the pregnancy for revealing the sex, I sent the intended mother a message on WhatsApp that I'd let her know the results. She replied, "We already know, it's a boy and a girl. No one told you?" I was sad. From that point, the relationship changed. Apparently they had paid extra to get a boy and a girl but my ultrasound showed I was having twin boys. The girl embryo that had been transferred was lost and the boy embryo twinned. The couple was very annoyed and kept asking everyone if this was true and what happened and who messed up. They were not happy. After that our relationship went from bad to worse!

My stress level escalated because of how they were treating me. When I would message them, trying to keep them updated on the pregnancy, they would tell me they were really busy and didn't have time.

After Christmas, I was about 28–29 weeks and I just didn't feel well. I had gained about 20 pounds in a week and I felt like something was wrong. I went to the hospital and had my blood pressure checked. It was very high and they monitored it for a few hours. The agency didn't want to contact the couple because they didn't want to worry them. They finally let me go home. At my next Ob appointment I had gained 30 pounds in one week. They did lab tests and my blood work was so bad they admitted me to the hospital straight away. I didn't contact the couple as I had received a message from the intended father that I was stressing his wife out!

I was already preparing to put the boys up for adoption since this couple was so mad about having two boys. Even my doctor said he and I needed a game plan since we weren't sure what this couple would do.

At 29 weeks I had severe pre-eclampsia and my kidneys and liver were shutting down. The couple finally arrived from Spain and when they walked into my room, the first thing they asked the doctor was "two boys?" The doctor ordered an ultrasound right then to show the couple it was indeed two boys! By 30 weeks, I was having what I thought was heartburn and didn't feel real good. I was pacing in my room, lying on the floor and just didn't feel right. I knew something was wrong because I was having trouble seeing anything. I called for the nurses and they said to call my husband, but I couldn't even see the numbers on my phone to call him, so the nurses made the phone call.

The doctor said we had to deliver the babies right away or we all might die. My husband didn't get to the hospital in time to be with me for the C-section, so only the intended mother was with me. She just stood there and it was so awkward. She never said, "oh my, you might die" or "what can I do for you?" I delivered exactly at 30 weeks and this is significant because my contract said that I would receive full compensation if I carried to 30 weeks. The intended parents later accused me of delivering exactly 10 weeks early just so I would get all my money!

After the delivery, the nurses came to me and asked when the intended parents would be coming back because they had some new baby care questions for them. I didn't know and it broke my heart to learn that these babies spent most of their first day of life alone.

I was overwhelmed after the delivery and tried to get back on my feet. I had no paid maternity leave and I had lost income because I couldn't work for so many weeks. But I didn't worry about my medical bills being paid as there was an escrow account set up and I was instructed to send my bills there and they would be paid. But the bills started coming and they weren't being paid and these are expensive medical bills that are piling up and the debt collectors were coming after me to pay the bills. I didn't have the money to pay these bills. It was then that I found out that the couple had taken the babies and left the hospital and me with thousands and thousands of dollars of debt. I tried to get the agency to pay these bills for almost a year. As soon as I told the agency I was going to Spain with Jennifer Lahl, they paid all my bills within 24 hours. They clearly had the money, but were just trying not to have to pay them.

I remain incredibly unwell and I have been diagnosed with Post-traumatic Stress Disorder (PTSD). Two international couples have exploited me, lied to me, and have caused my family and me so much suffering. And all because I wanted to help them having a child in their lives.

Would I do surrogacy again or recommend this 'journey' to other women?

No, because the risk of harm is just too great, I almost died, and I put my children through a lot. I worry too about what's going to happen with the children I gave birth to.

Surrogacy Broke up Our Family
Rob (Australia)
Partner of a surrogate

I knew both Bev and Terri after meeting them at a work event. I never really liked Terri, or her husband Alex, who was known by everyone as 'The Sponge'.

It was only after I had known Bev for a year and a half that we got together as a couple at the end of 2011. This was after she had split from her husband Joe. It was at this time that I first learned about her plans to be a surrogate, which she had been putting into place while she was still married to Joe. She already had children, three boys aged 12, 7 and 4, and she really felt she wanted to help Terri and her husband to have a child of their own. Terri has a serious medical condition, so carrying a pregnancy was not possible for her health-wise with all the risks, and the couple's attempts at adoption were unsuccessful.

I said to Bev that I didn't have a problem with her being a surrogate, but I had a big problem with her being a surrogate for this particular couple. I knew them and didn't like them — they were users, and I didn't think they were trustworthy or would follow through on their promises. But she felt that she wanted to keep her word and help them.

Terri and Alex were also keen for the pregnancy to happen quickly. With Bev and me now a couple, that presented problems for them, because it would mean Bev and I would need to go through a thorough counselling process, as she had done previously with Joe. This would cause delays in getting the medical side of the surrogacy process underway. So their solution was to pretend I didn't exist. I was 'a secret'. The couple lied to the IVF clinic in Melbourne, which required compulsory counselling with your partner before surrogacy could go ahead. By pretending I didn't exist, Bev was considered a single mother and the birth process could go ahead and stay on schedule. It was all about what Terri and Alex wanted.

When Bev started the medical procedures, such as progesterone treatment, things went downhill quickly. Terri and Alex insisted that Bev and I could not have sex, even protected sex. We felt like they were overstepping the mark, trying to tell us how to live. It was especially hard as we were a new couple and this was really intruding on our own relationship.

The first IVF transfer did not work. The second IVF transfer ended in a miscarriage at seven weeks. The third IVF transfer worked and Bev did become pregnant with an embryo using an egg donor and Alex's sperm. You would think that with Bev now pregnant, and her supporting her own three young boys, all the promises Terri and Alex had made would kick in, given that she was expecting their child. But as I had feared, all the talk about helping her out came to nothing.

Bev was often sick during the pregnancy and needed lots of help with cooking, washing and housework. She suffered from severe morning sickness and at one time ended up in hospital for the day. Terri and Alex lived five minutes away from her but did absolutely nothing. For the entire length of her pregnancy, the only things they did were, on one occasion only, to wash Bev's car, and one other time, to cook a meal. They would drive her to her ante-natal appointments. But the appointments were all about the baby. They did not care or show any concern about Bev and her acute morning sickness. Instead it was me who had to drop everything and help Bev. I lived on the other side of the city at the time, and also had a four-year-old son of my own who needed me around. After work, I would come home and attend to my son and things that would have to be done at home, and then most nights I was driving to Bev's place on the other side of the city to help her with the housework, cooking, cleaning and doing things like making the boys' lunches for school. I used up all my sick leave and annual leave to help Bev out as she had no one else. It was exhausting for me and terrible for Bev who felt so let down by Terri and Alex and the empty promises they had made.

During her pregnancy, Bev also had to move house. Terri and Alex had known about this in advance, and had promised to help her, but it too came to nothing.

Bev had also been promised money to buy maternity clothes. It never eventuated. She had called Terri one morning to say that she needed to buy maternity clothes, but she could not get hold of her. So she spent $350 on clothes which included maternity bras, shorts, t-shirts and cardigans. Terri and Alex became extremely angry that she had spent this money. However, around the same time, Terri had a christening to attend for a friend in Queensland. She was happy to spend money on a new outfit, new shoes, airfares and accommodation, and getting her nails and hair done. Terri and Alex were happy to look after themselves, but not their surrogate. At one point they offered Bev used hand-me-down maternity clothes from a cousin of theirs who was a totally different size. How insulting! Instead I gave Bev money so she could buy the clothes she urgently needed.

As Bev's pregnancy continued, things only got worse. From day one Terri and Alex had promised that one of them would babysit and look after Bev's children while she gave birth and after the birth while she was in hospital. It was getting to six weeks before her due date when Terri and Alex told Bev that they couldn't babysit the kids because they both wanted to be present at the birth. Bev had never agreed to this and so she said to them "I have babysat your baby for nine months in my belly, so you can babysit my children for five days while I give birth and recover from having your baby."

One day, while Bev was still pregnant, Terri and Alex came to the house. I was there too, as were the children. Terri and Alex were totally abusive, which resulted in a huge argument. Alex then drove around and around the block, circling the house. This culminated with Alex banging on the door and screaming, "You have my baby so you do as I say!" Both of them had no care or concern for Bev's welfare at all. It was all about them and their child. Alex spent that night out the front of Bev's house in his car. It was like stalking her.

After this argument, some vandalism occurred, including damage to my car and garden stakes being thrown at the house. We don't have firm evidence it was them, but I am pretty sure it was. The situation was getting out of control.

Yet despite this awful build-up, Bev, against my advice, decided to still allow Terri and Alex into the birthing suite when the baby was born at the hospital in November 2012. Terri and Alex were meant to take it in turns looking after Bev's youngest son while the other was in the birthing suite. But Terri left Bev's youngest son alone with a nurse and snuck into the birthing room while Bev was trying to push the baby out. This made Bev very distressed wondering where her son was and who was looking after him.

The birth was not too difficult, but we didn't get any time at all with the baby after she was born. The couple whisked her off into another hospital room that they had booked for themselves. The five minutes after her birth is the only time Bev and I have spent with her daughter, with Terri in the room supervising. It was enough to take a photo, and that was it.

I posted on social media the news that the birth had gone well and that Bev was okay. When Alex found that out, he was verbally abusive to me. Even at this time, his concern was about them, and keeping up the pretence that they had a baby without another woman being involved. It was like me mentioning Bev spoiled the mirage of them telling the world about their baby. As far as they were concerned, it was only their news to tell and Bev was just a means to an end, not a person in her own right.

This was drummed home to us as Alex and Terri received an endless succession of relatives and friends visiting them in their hospital room. Not a single one inquired about how Bev was, or popped in to see her and check on her welfare.

In fact, by staying at the hospital, Alex was reneging on yet another agreement. I was staying with Bev in the hospital and it had been agreed beforehand that Alex would go to Bev's house to look after her three boys as there was no one else. He tried to get out of this, too. But I stood my ground and insisted on staying with Bev in the hospital.

Alex eventually went to mind the boys, but we found out later that the day of the birth, he dropped the boys at home and left them unattended while he went home to drink alcohol before coming back to the boys. He had left them alone without adult supervision for an hour and a half.

Bev completed her recovery at a hotel, which is common nowadays with maternity patients. When we returned to her house we were really upset to learn that Alex had looked after the children while drunk. The entire liquor cabinet was emptied of all it contents. There was not a drop of anything left.

The hospital stay was made even worse by the fact that the bill for Bev's hospital bed was left unpaid and it was in Bev's name. Terri and Alex paid $1000 a night for a hospital room for them to stay in with the baby once it was born because they were not patients themselves. They stayed with the baby for three nights which cost them $3000, but refused to pay an extra $68 so Bev could have a double bed room in order for me to stay with her after she had given birth and provide her with support. It turned out to be yet another broken promise and we were stuck with the bill when Bev was discharged.

The little girl that was born was called Rebecca. Bev had been promised her middle name would be Sue which is Bev's middle name. You won't be surprised to learn that commitment was broken too.

Besides those five minutes in the hospital, the only other time we have seen Rebecca was in court for the parentage order, which granted parentage rights to Terri and Alex. Bev is named as the mother on the birth certificate. I, of course, am totally hidden from the whole thing as if I didn't exist. Bev had to appear at court on her own for the parentage order, because she could not afford for the unpaid legal bills to get any higher. Terri and Alex had stopped paying legal fees for her, even though this was part of the agreement too.

Bev was promised she would be known as an aunty and the godmother to the baby, and have the chance to see her and watch her grow up as aunts do. Instead she has not spent any time with her and only seen her on those two occasions: five minutes in hospital, and glimpsing her across the courtroom where she was used as a prop by Terri and Alex to help their case.

The last few years have been a relentless process of legal proceedings. Bev and I have been trying to recover the costs incurred from her being a surrogate, including the hospital expenses and legal costs. We have got back some, but not all of what we spent.

The surrogacy-related expenses that Bev was asking for were not a great amount, considering she carried a child for them for nine months. It was a list of the following:

1. $55 for travel expenses to and from a doctor's appointment on 19 November;
2. $55 for travel expenses to and from the hospital on 26 November and 30 November;
3. $189 for post-pregnancy recovery shorts;
4. $68 for carparking at the hospital (Terri and Alex refused to pay this because I drove Bev in my car while she was in labour and they expected her to catch a taxi which would have cost more money.);
5. Bev's legal costs;
6. $55 for travel expenses to and from an obstetric appointment at the hospital on 27 December;
7. $55 for travel expenses to and from an obstetric appointment at the hospital on 13 January;
8. hotel room service dinner meals for the kids, Bev and me totalling $184.73. (We kept a text message that Terri sent Bev saying that she would pay for our meals as proof. She later lied and stated that she was not covering this cost.)

The relationship between Terri, Alex and us has deteriorated further since the time of Rebecca's birth. Terri and Bev now have five-year intervention orders out against each other. Terri has hacked into Bev's social media accounts, spreading false rumours about her. She has made prank calls, and had false reports made about Bev to Centrelink. She has harrassed her online and encouraged others to do the same. No wonder Bev has struggled since the birth of the baby.

There was an agreement between Bev, Terri and Alex that Bev would only be a surrogate if she could give birth in a private hospital of her choice with an obstetrician of her choice. They agreed to this arrangement during counselling sessions with the IVF clinic. I wanted this for Bev too because I wanted her to have the best medical care as she was putting her life on the line to have this baby. On 31 January 2013 Bev received a letter from her private health insurance stating that her nominated financial institution had declined their most recent attempt to debit her premium. The bank account that was to be debited was in Terri and Alex's name. The insurance premium was left $259.93 in arrears. When Bev rang up the insurance company, they stated that Terri had tried to cancel the policy but wasn't able to because the insurance policy was in Bev's name. So Terri rang up her bank and cancelled the direct debit. Terri and Alex did not advise Bev that they were going to do this. They did not even check with Bev that she was medically okay after the birth or whether she still needed the health insurance in case there were complications after the surrogacy. The letter came days before her son's birthday and, after paying the lapsed premium, she did not have enough money to buy him a gift. This was just vindictive, nasty and spiteful on Terri's and Alex's part.

On 14 January, Terri made hurtful comments about Bev on a Facebook group which supports those who want to become parents through the use of surrogacy arrangements. Terri posted that Bev had become severely resentful and mentally unstable and refused to sign the birth certificate and parentage order. She stated that the IVF counsellors were trying to persuade her to sign, which was untrue.

She posted that Bev's demands while she was pregnant became ridiculous, like mowing her lawns and doing housework.

The truth is that Bev had already signed the birth registration statement which allows a birth certificate to be issued, which was being held by her lawyer, but Bev was not intending to sign the parentage order until all her out-of-pocket expenses were paid, including her legal costs. Not signing the parentage order was the only hope she had of recovering costs that were owed to her.

On the Facebook page, Terri also posted private medical information about Bev, telling everyone she had pre-natal depression during pregnancy and saw a psychiatrist. It was true that during the pregnancy Bev was finding it hard to manage without any help coming from Terri and Alex. On top of that, her own mum was extremely sick and in palliative care. She died when Bev was 34 weeks pregnant. But Terri posted about the depression in a way to humiliate Bev and to paint a picture that she was unstable. Terri also falsified her court statement saying that Bev had tried to "induce abortion" and kill the baby when pregnant and that Bev believed that the baby was hers.

On the 16 March 2014, Terri created a new Facebook account in her name and sent Facebook friend requests to Bev and her two eldest children. I found these attempts of contact strange considering all the nasty things Terri had previously posted about Bev on Facebook. It was just another form of harassment and stalking. Terri and Alex were advised by Bev's lawyer that she did not want them to contact her children without her consent.

On the 16 May, Bev was signed up to hundreds of religious mailing lists that had flooded her email inbox. Bev is not religious and it was obvious that Terri had organised this as another form of harassment, as one of the mailing lists had stated the internet address used to sign her up. Police later confirmed that it was Terri who had done this.

Also on the 16 May, I was signed up to the Ashley Madison website, which is a website to have discreet sexual affairs. My personal information was used and I believe that Terri and Alex were behind this.

On the 17 May, Bev received an email from the ANZ bank stating that a credit card had been applied for in her name, however it was refused because the driver's licence number was incorrect. Bev and I went to the police station and an investigation was conducted. We told the police that we believed it was Terri and Alex. We also passed on the IP address from the religious emails to the police. It was Terri and Alex's IP address. This gave the police enough evidence to get a search warrant and take their electronic equipment. There was no proof on their computers that they applied for the credit card. However, I still believe it was them and that they used a friend's computer or a portable device.

On 3 August, I received a friend request from a woman named Daisy who stated that Bev is a 'psycho mum' and her children hate her. It also said that it would be really funny to see Bev's passport taken off her. I believe Terri and Alex were behind this as well. They knew that we were going on a holiday to California as it was mentioned in a lawyer's letter regarding court dates for parentage orders. They were trying to upset our travel plans.

Bev sent a letter to the judge before the parentage order was made because she did not want the judge to be misled. She made it clear that her legal costs and expenses had not been paid, and she was harrassed and stalked, especially online and on Facebook forums.

Emotionally, Bev is up and down. It has been made so much worse by the fact that the court ordered that Bev cannot talk about Terri or about Rebecca. Not being able to talk openly about her experience of being a surrogate means that Bev has been effectively silenced. How can she possibly process and come to terms with this traumatic experience when she can't even talk freely about it?

She has attempted suicide and has struggled to cope as we have faced financial, legal and emotional hurdles. Life has been really hard. As of 10 May, both Bev and Terri have further 5-year intervention orders against each other and their children. But there is no sign that the trouble and harrassment will end, as despite Terri and Alex now being recognised as parents, Terri is still jealous of Bev, who had the child that she could never have. Instead of being grateful and keeping her promises, Terri puts Bev down online to others while finding her own allies among other parents like her. We feel totally used and betrayed.

Surrogacy broke up our family at the very time we were trying to establish it. Instead of having her three sons around her, and an extra baby girl to watch grow up, Bev lost one son who went to live with his father and we never see the girl she gave birth to. The toll on us all has been enormous.

Even now Terri has created a disgusting Instagram account with the sole purpose of mocking Bev's mental illness (she has been diagnosed with PTSD) and saying her whole life is fake — baby, husband, everything — belittling and dismissing Bev's experiences.

This is what surrogacy has brought to our family: a cycle of destruction and despair that we can only hope will end. But will it?

My Heart Is Hurting
Ujwala, Dimpy and Sarala (India)

As told by Sheela Saravanan

I collected the following stories of so-called surrogate mothers as part of my ethnographic research in India from 2009 to 2010 (published as *A Transnational Feminist View of Surrogacy Biomarkets in India*, 2018). I was based at two IVF clinics in Gujarat and was able to talk with surrogate mothers and intending parents. In 2016, India passed the Surrogacy (Regulation) Bill that in theory prohibits surrogacy for foreigners. At the time of writing (September 2018), the Bill has still not been fully implemented.

I have become friends with the Indian women and we stayed in touch over the years. As background to their stories it is important to know that in many cases, surrogate mothers are expected to stay in dormitory accommodations called 'surrogate homes' where beds are lined up 'hostel style' in the rooms. The women's movements are restricted; I saw them even prevented from using the staircase or the elevator by themselves – this was only allowed with the assistance of nurses or other hospital personnel. The women are not supposed to do any work. They are overfed in the hope that this might increase the birth weight of the child for which the clinic will be paid extra money, but the food is very poor quality. Their family and children are allowed to visit them only on Sundays, under restrictive conditions such as their children must not sit on their bed. There is also a restriction on the kind of music they are allowed to listen to; for instance, they are expected to listen to *Bhajans* (religious songs) because this is said to have a positive impact on the unborn child. After the birth of the child(ren), they are expected to provide breastmilk and 'nanny care' according to the requirement of the intended parents.

It is these rules, the lack of rights and the 'cheap' prices for surrogacy that attract 'intended mothers' like Caroline from Canada to India for surrogacy. In what follows I describe the experiences of three surrogate mothers in contracting out their bodily rights over their unique physiological, emotional and creative capacity of growing and giving birth to a baby. I tell the stories of Ujwala and Caroline, Dimpy and her husband Dhiraj, and Sarala, who I followed during their pregnancies and relinquishment processes. Ujwala was a surrogate mother of twins born for Caroline from Canada, Dimpy gave birth to a baby girl born for a heterosexual couple from Turkey. Sarala, Dimpy's sister in law, was a surrogate mother to twins born for Indian intended parents. (All names are pseudonyms.)

Ujwala and Caroline

Ujwala was a domestic worker living on the edge of poverty. With her husband and one child they rented a one-room house without bathroom and toilet. With her money from the surrogacy she wanted to buy a similar house that had these amenities. She also hoped to save money for her eight-year-old son's education.

The intended mother, Caroline, worked as a human resource professional for a company in Canada. She had adopted her first child from Vietnam but continued to be very distressed, as she wanted at least one child that looked German. Her husband of German origin owned a computer firm in Canada. They used her husband's sperm and her friend's egg cell for the surrogacy. She selected this particular Indian clinic because they do not charge any major payment until the baby is handed over. Caroline had been satisfied that the surrogate mother was paid nominal instalments throughout the pregnancy with a final lump sum only after the child was handed over: *"It [small instalments] keeps her motivated to carry on with the pregnancy."*

The surrogate mothers in this clinic were paid US$30 per month and US$6400 at the end. Caroline commented that, *"Although surrogacy is legal in my country, the process is very complex and much more expensive than [in] India. The law expects surrogate mothers in India to sign over all rights to the baby even before the surrogacy begins, which is a big relief ... I am also happy that she [the surrogate mother] was monitored throughout the pregnancy, her food and everyday life during the pregnancy was taken care of."* It is clear that Caroline had come to India because surrogate mothers have fewer rights over the baby. In her description of surrogate mothers, she constructed them as objects, as risky and unclean bodies to be medically monitored, maintained and controlled during the pregnancy.

Ujwala gave birth to twins (one girl and one boy) and Caroline was very happy that the boy child had the phenotype she desired. Because the children's passport application process took a while, Caroline wanted Ujwala to look after the babies. While Caroline stayed in one hotel room, Ujwala and the children stayed in the adjoining room. Ujwala was expected to breastfeed the children and provide nanny services along with another caretaker appointed by Caroline. She was upset that the children were responding more to Ujwala than to her own voice: *"When I say something, they do not respond to me, but when Ujwala says something in her pitched tone, they immediately respond to her. They seem to be more comfortable with her."* I also observed that Caroline went to the children's room only to see if they needed anything or to accompany Ujwala when the children had to be taken to the clinic for check-ups. The interactions were always between Caroline and Ujwala; Caroline's husband only came once to India to deposit his sperm for the IVF process.

On the day of the relinquishment of the twins, Ujwala said, *"I am happy to have given life to these children and [I] have to give them [the children] away as a gift [to this couple] though my heart is hurting* (she shuddered as she said this). *These children are part of my life but the deal [the contract] was made right at the beginning and I have to keep it up by giving them away."* The baby starts to cry during this conversation and she puts him on her shoulder and with gentle pats tries to quieten him. When I asked Caroline about Ujwala's emotions on giving the baby away, she said, *"I'm not sure if the surrogates or doctor at the clinic themselves would ever use the phrase 'give the baby away.' These words are usually introduced by the media and the people who interview them."* On being asked about bonding between the surrogate mother and the twins, Caroline's comment was that, *"From the very beginning the doctors try to counsel the surrogate in a way that makes her aware that the baby(s) are not hers to 'give away' and that they result from embryos belonging to the biological parents."* The clinic's doctor, Dr Nisha also spoke along the same lines. She told me that the surrogate mothers are well aware that the child does not belong to them and that they are only renting their womb temporarily to another couple who would then take the child(ren) that rightfully belong to them.

I stayed in touch with Caroline after she had arrived with the babies in Canada. The girl had gotten used to the changes, but the boy was very restless: *"It can be very difficult to get him to stop crying; when the crying really escalates, he becomes apoplectic."* Caroline complained about not having enough assistance. She had not found a nanny, and was struggling with the children for several months until she found a young Filipino woman who was dedicated and managed well with the children. Regarding the impact of the relinquishment on the surrogate mother after bonding and breastfeeding for several months, Caroline said, *"I am told that some doctors recommend that the surrogate should not spend too much time with the baby(s) after they are born to help minimize the pain of separation. In fact, our reasons for inviting Ujwala to spend so much time with us was really to help me tend to our babies through provision of breast milk and extra baby minding. As she was obliging, our reasons could be considered selfish by some and while we also had an interest in getting to know her better and developing a relationship, sometimes I wonder if we did her a disservice."*

The doctor in the clinic knew that after the surrogacy, Ujwala was still short of the money needed to buy a house. Although Caroline wanted to pay her extra, the clinic staff stopped her from doing so and commented, *"Don't spoil our surrogate mothers – then they become greedy."* The reality is that they wanted Ujwala to return for another surrogacy so they could make more money from her body. Caroline never visited Ujwala's house; she had Ujwala's phone number and contact details, but had not given her own contact number to Ujwala. According to Ujwala, this distance was maintained by Caroline because of the fear created by the doctors who portrayed surrogate mothers and their family members as 'money-grabbers' and 'blackmailers'. Caroline sent messages and photos to my email address and I then visited Ujwala and gave her the children's photos. When I went to Ujwala's house she posed for a photo with her son and the photo of the twins. She considered this to be her only photo with all her children.

The relationship between Caroline and Ujwala was clearly not of two equals and nowhere near the 'global sisterhood' concept emphasised by some gender researchers (e.g. Amrita Pande, Sharmila Rudrappa). Ujwala bonded with the children and although Caroline felt she may have been doing a disservice to Ujwala, she continued to maintain the unequal relationship because it suited her. This case reveals that filiation and genetic ties are given precedence over the gestational role. Caroline felt an ownership over the children because she had selected/bought the gametes for the surrogacy. She also felt she had control over Ujwala's body and services as she had commissioned and was paying for every aspect of the surrogacy (IVF, food, accommodation, gestation and nanny services) and the children. Additionally, she also paid for Ujwala's nursing course and deposited some money for her son's education. These are indications of a form of *recolonisation* over biomaterials (bodies, gametes, embryos, and children).

Dimpy (and her husband Dhiraj)

After several days of waiting at the clinic to meet more surrogate mothers, one day Dr Harnish (the assistant of Dr Nisha) asked if I would like to meet a surrogate mother who was staying at the children's hospital along with the baby she gave birth to. He informed the children's hospital that I would be visiting. There, I heard about tensions regarding the Turkish parents because they were out of contact and had not arrived from Turkey despite information that the child was born.

Dimpy and Dhiraj were agricultural labourers from a neighbouring rural area. Sarala (Dimpy's sister-in-law), who was also considering surrogacy, was working in a hospital as a nursing assistant. But Sarala was scared of the surrogacy process and did not want to go alone into the surrogate home. She convinced her brother Dhiraj to send his wife along with her to become a surrogate. It took Dimpy two attempts to conceive. She gave birth to a baby girl and they were shifted to a nearby children's hospital.

I asked the doctor why she had left the baby with Dimpy to which she replied, *"Who else can I entrust the baby other than the surrogate mother?"* Dr Nisha had earlier told me that surrogate mothers only want the money and have no interest in the baby and don't (want to) bond with the child. But what I saw at the children's hospital when I went to meet Dimpy after the delivery was very different. Dimpy's attachment to the child was evident in her affectionate kissing and fondling, either in response to the baby's distressed cries or during play time. She told me that she had started breastfeeding just naturally as the baby was with her all the time. She and Dhiraj were changing nappies and providing all the required care for the child. The couple had even named the child Amita (also their younger daughter's name).

I became very fond of little Amita as I spent more and more time with them. They were very hopeful that the couple would want to keep in further contact with them. After 21 days, the intended parents arrived from Turkey with gifts for Dimpy. But as per the rule of the clinic, they handed over the money to the doctor and then left without meeting her again. Dimpy was heartbroken when she came to know that they had been in the same building but didn't come to say goodbye. Dhiraj was very happy with the payment but Dimpy was clearly disinterested in the money or the counting of it, though she was happy that her husband was happy. Dhiraj categorically told us (myself and Dimpy) never to utter this baby's name (Amita) ever again. That didn't resolve the depression that Dimpy was experiencing. She was distressed that her children at home would never be able to meet Amita. In another incident, when I was taking photos of them and myself, and Dimpy was reviewing the photos, I mistakenly scrolled on to Amita's photo. Although she didn't say anything, her expression revealed the emotional turmoil she was going through.

Sarala

Dimpy and Dhiraj asked me to visit their village a week after they returned so that people would not get suspicious that they were involved in surrogacy. They had not informed their extended family about the surrogacy. It was Sarala (Dhiraj's sister) who took me to Dimpy's village. Sarala worked as a nurse and earned Rs 900 (US$12.50) per month. Her husband worked as a gardener in a Christian mission and his salary varied. Some months they paid him all the arrears together and other times he was not paid at all. Sarala came to know of surrogacy through some friends. She was unable to convince her husband that this would be a good option for her to earn a lot of money. She then persuaded her brother Dhiraj and through him his wife Dimpy to go along with her to the surrogate home. Both women set out to earn money through surrogacy. Both went to the clinic together, went through the initial clearance and met the respective intended parents. However, Sarala became pregnant at the first attempt for a couple and remained at the surrogate home, while Dimpy was unsuccessful and had to return home only to join her again a few months later. Sarala's intended parents were non-resident Indians (NRIs), originally from Rajasthan. She received Rs 350,000 (US$4,800) for the surrogacy. Sarala has three children, two daughters and one son. She had left her two children in the hostel of the Christian mission for a year because her husband was unable to look after them at home and her mother-in-law refused to care for them. She was worried about their well-being but couldn't go to meet them although she was staying in a surrogacy home very close to her own home.

She described her surrogacy experience as follows: *"This process is so distressing that I would not have done it even if someone paid me ten times the remuneration, had I been well-off. But I am so desperate [for money] that I would do it even if I was paid just one third the amount."* She was allowed to come home for festivals only because she had a good relationship with the matron. Her sister-in-law, Dimpy, joined her at the surrogate home after a few months. Her brother and her husband would visit them every weekend and bring them some home food. Sarala resisted intermediary power such as the dormitory matron and tried her best within the home to improve the food and facilities. She said the only time they cleaned the dormitory well was when a TV documentary crew came with cameras. 'Intended parents' never came to this dormitory as it was situated around 20 km away from the clinic. Sarala said the food provided was sub-standard although the intended parents paid Rs 6000 (US$83) per month for each surrogate mother for this purpose and there were at least ten women housed at this dormitory at the same time. On enquiring about the food, the matron would say, *"At least here you are eating two full meals a day and not just the Baakhri [unleavened bread made of millet flour] and green chilies that you get at home so be happy with whatever we give you."* Sarala complained about the food to Dr Nisha but it was to no avail. Sarala, however, told me never to disclose what she had told me to Dr Nisha, as she now works for the clinic as a so-called surrogate 'agent' (i.e. recruiting other women to become surrogates for a commission).

Sarala' s husband complained that the intended parents could not be bothered and never tried to find out about what was happening in the dormitory homes. He opined that they should take more care of what the surrogate mother eats and in what condition she lives.

Sarala said that some of the cash and other gifts that were sent by the intended parents were generally pocketed by the matron. Phone calls from intended parents were not passed on to surrogate mothers in order to keep control over the relationship. Sarala gave birth to twins, one boy and one girl, and she showed me their photographs. Both were grossly underweight, which is quite usual, as the women are often anaemic, in poor health and fed poor quality food. Overall, Sarala had a bad experience with the intended parents after birth. She tended to the babies as the parents arrived late and she was breastfeeding the children. After the parents came and took the babies to their hotel, Sarala too left for home without waiting for payment. She was eager to see her children and husband who had been without her for a year. After a week, she called the parents and requested to see the babies and they agreed. They asked her to wait at the clinic in the evening where they would bring the babies. She waited there patiently expecting them to come. She even called them twice and she was assured that they would bring the children but they never came. She waited with her son hoping that he would get to see the babies she had borne but returned home very late at night, feeling dejected. As in many other cases, the parents never called her to enquire about her or ensure the well-being of her other children. The behaviour of the intended parents changed from kindness (during pregnancy) to neglect (after relinquishment). This was observed by all surrogate mothers. Sarala remarked, *"In a way it is good that they are not in touch, otherwise I would have asked for the children to be returned."*

In India (and elsewhere), surrogate mothers are coached by their medical practitioners to believe that the child genetically belongs to someone else and that she is merely offering her uterus – an empty room in her body – for carrying the baby to term. In the documentary film *Made in India,* Dr Kaushul Kadam from the Rotunda Clinic said, *"I educate these surrogates. I say 'I'm going to prepare a baby outside and put it into their uterus.' I tell them I only need their uterus."*

Separating gestation and childbirth from the rest of a woman's being is a form of alienation. Despite all the coaching and reminding by the medical practitioners to distance themselves from their womb, the surrogate mothers in India that I interviewed explained their relationship with the children as motherhood, blood relations, and siblings to their existing children. Shama, a surrogate mother in my study emphasised, *"I am the mother of the child, I have carried the baby. They may have given the genetic material but I have given the blood to the child. Whatever I consume the child also eats, I'm carrying the baby for nine months, so this will have some effect on me."* The surrogate mothers also want to maintain a long-lasting relationship, especially to be reassured about the well-being of the children. But the doctors at the IVF clinics tell the intended parents that surrogate mothers do not want to bond with the children; they only want the money. These lies are used to control the women and commodify their birth children, which amounts to human rights violations. The only solution is to abolish the practice of surrogacy worldwide, as regulation will never work.

Messing with My Body, Messing with My Mind
Marie Anne (UK)

"Can you help me?" This is the question that changed my life forever. Regrets – without a shadow of a doubt, I have regrets. My story is written with one sole purpose in mind – to ensure that no one ever suffers like I have from exploitation via the use of surrogacy.

I entered a gestational surrogacy arrangement on trust alone with no contract in place – a huge mistake. The current situation in the UK is such that surrogacy contracts are not enforceable. But at least a contract would have clarified my position and given me something tangible to later argue my case in the courts.

I believed that by helping my cousin to have her baby, I would enrich not only her life, but the lives of others as well. How wrong I was. I asked for three conditions to be met. First, that my health would be their priority. Second, that my children would always be my priority, and finally, that I would have contact with the child that I was to give birth to. "Of course," was the response I was given. "We are family – there is trust," I was told.

That was not to be the case. Eventually I was to lose my physical and mental health. And even my children.

Growing up, my cousin and I were extremely close. Her father and my father are brothers. We were in each other's lives from when we were toddlers until I had her baby. She was even chief bridesmaid at my wedding.

Unfortunately, my cousin had her womb removed due to cancer treatment when she was 35. But before this, she had the foresight to have embryos frozen. Asking me to be a gestational surrogate for her seemed like a simple proposition. As it is illegal to be paid for surrogacy in the UK, my cousin attempted to pay me by offering to buy a new kitchen for my house. I declined this offer and told her I was doing this for love. I also made it clear that I was very much against commercial surrogacy.

But what I did not take into account was the resentment that arose from me being able to do the one thing she so desperately wanted to do herself: to carry a baby. This resentment was never spoken about. Instead of admitting to it, talking through her feelings and getting counselling, she denied it and continued to deny it even after the birth. By now, I am exhausted with trying to understand what went on in my cousin's head back then. This is about saving me and my family.

All through the pregnancy there were complications. Due to the hormone treatment, I suffered extreme sickness, which lasted from when I woke up until I went to sleep. For the first three months of pregnancy these hormonal drugs consisted of a high dose of progesterone and blood thinners to stop blood clots. I had not been told of any potential risks to my health.

Once I was pregnant I was also pressured to agree to an abortion in the event the child was diagnosed with an abnormality. My cousin, her partner and I had never talked about this before. Similarly I was pressured to have a C-Section, again something we had never discussed before the pregnancy. I was able to avoid having a C-Section though with the help of my midwife who made it very clear that it was not necessary and was not in the best interests of my health nor the child's. A consultant with the hospital did try to change my mind but I insisted that the only way I would have a C-Section was if my life or the child's life was in danger.

In the UK, parental consent must be obtained by the intended parents whereby legally the birth mother relinquishes her rights to the child. After the child was born I refused to give parental consent to people I no longer trusted. As a consequence my cousin and her partner took me to court. In the end I was bullied and intimidated by the couple into signing away all my parental rights in a British Court of Law. This led to a complete breakdown in my mental health.

Then, to make matters even worse, without my consent, pictures of my womb were plastered all over a tabloid newspaper! That's right: pictures of my womb, taken from an ultrasound during my pregnancy, were given to a newspaper by my cousin, so that she could tell the world what a lucky person she was for having survived cancer and having a baby. She also used this publicity to advertise her own new fertility business, which included surrogacy services.

In other words, not only had I been used to have a baby for her, but she then used this baby to make money.

Not surprisingly, my health was badly affected by the hormonal changes due to the fertility drugs I had taken during the pregnancy, but also from the emotional upheaval of the surrogacy itself and the dreadful way in which I was treated by my cousin including being dragged to court. There are days when I truly do not understand how I continue to survive.

Does a woman carrying a child in her womb, whether it is her baby or not, develop feelings for it? The answer I am sure varies from person to person. For me, at the start, I didn't have strong feelings for the baby because I knew on an intellectual level it was not my egg, so therefore I thought it was not my 'genetic' child. I did not feel the same way about this baby growing inside me as I had when pregnant with my own children. But that didn't mean I didn't care for the baby, and it didn't mean I didn't want to protect the baby.

However, my feelings of attachments did grow stronger as the pregnancy went on. After the birth there was numbness in me. There was a void and I had no support. I told myself, "Do what they want. Do what everyone says. Forget about your own intense feelings." I remember not being allowed to express remorse or sorrow for a natural loss of this child. I received no advice or counselling on how to deal with my feelings of attachment to the baby. I sought advice on the internet and tried to draw from my previous experience with my own pregnancies.

Clinics don't provide surrogate mothers with information or emotional or physical support when they become attached to the babies they carry; they only seemed interested in talking about the physical risks associated with pregnancy and childbirth. The same was true of my cousin who didn't wish to discuss my feelings about anything during or after the pregnancy.

My own children were far more resilient than me at the time, but later I realised that the surrogacy psychologically affected my daughter as well. For a long time, she couldn't say the word 'baby' and turned off television programmes that showed babies on them either to protect her or me – or both of us. The surrogacy was also a terrible process for my partner who, by his own admission, had no feelings for this baby. But he saw, and had to deal with, the emotional fallout from it all. And he had to care for our children when I couldn't do it any more. He had to give up his work when it became too much for me, which meant financial devastation for us.

My baby was born in May 2014 and one year after the birth, I was told by a psychologist that I suffer from Post-Traumatic Stress Disorder, as well as Post-Partum Psychosis. None of this was picked up after the baby was born. Even now, I continue to suffer from severe mood swings, which can range from moderate depression to suicidal thoughts. Anxiety and panic attacks occur daily and both my children and I have had to receive counselling. I also have an enlarged uterus and had a biopsy to find out why this is the case. My concern is that the hormone treatments I was subjected to during the surrogacy have played a role in this problem. All of these health problems are the results of the stress and anxiety of the surrogacy, including the combination of fertility drugs I was given, and how I was treated during the pregnancy and in its aftermath.

Things became so bad that my children's father brought the matter to the courts, along with evidence from Social Services that my health was posing a risk to my children's welfare and they were all concerned about my state of mind. In October 2015, my children, then aged eleven and seven, were removed from my care to live with my ex-husband, their father, who I had divorced before the surrogacy. (My current partner had no say in the matter. Luckily all this stress did not divide us as a couple.) Removing my own children was certainly not going to help me when I was already grieving the loss of the child I delivered for my cousin. Thankfully, my children have now been returned to my care but their removal from me for nearly a year caused me additional trauma and great distress.

I worked as a teacher before all of this, and now my career has ended. I cannot bring myself any longer to care for anybody else's children, other than my own.

I fervently believe that no woman should ever be paid for having a baby – nobody has the right to buy a child no matter the circumstances. But even if no money is involved, surrogacy comes with insurmountable risks and problems – look what happened to my life.

I wonder how my cousin and her partner can be so cruel and inhumane, knowing that I am still suffering with enormous distress and psychological torture, when I am the one person they should be grateful to. I asked for an apology – it took many attempts to get one and the words were, "We are sorry you feel that we have caused you hurt and upset." Why do two people find it so difficult to take responsibility for the damage they have caused? Do they feel guilt? Are they in denial? Do they have a hidden sense of remorse? I don't know. They even indicated to me in the court proceedings that they regret I am their child's birth mother. I am sure this is because they resent the fact that I gave birth to their daughter, the one thing my cousin could not do. They will never admit this though. And they dare not ask me if I regret the surrogacy. I think they know what the answer is.

My daughter asked me what she should do if somebody asked her to have a baby for them. My answer was simple. "Say no. You can't mess with your body and your mind like that. Not for anybody."

Surrogacy Is Business
Elena (Romania)

As told to Eva Maria Bachinger[5]

It's a drizzly day in Bucharest, Romania. I am 15 minutes early and wait between a bank and a fast food restaurant in a busy shopping centre in downtown Bucharest. In one way it's strange to meet a surrogate mother in a shopping centre, but in another it's quite apt. Arranging a surrogacy is business: carrying a pregnancy with a resulting child for money. All of a sudden a tall blond woman emerges from the grey mass of people rushing past me. She has a bow draped over her hair like a little girl. I look at her somewhat irritatedly. In her hand she has one of those flyers from shops that offer 25% discount on the whole stock. "Hi, I am Elena," she says in almost accent-free British-sounding English.

When I turned 32, I was desperate to have a baby. I was overdue to become a mother. I wanted to be pregnant, get fat and round, be able to breastfeed, finally not to be useless anymore. Almost out of desperation, because that whole partner-and-baby-thing was still not working, a few months ago I registered as a potential surrogate mother on the website <findsurrogate.com>. Within a few days I received inquiries from around the world. I speak very good English and type fast and without mistakes, but even my fingers were not quick enough to send an answer to everyone. They wrote to me from

---

5 I conducted this interview for my 2015 book *Kind auf Bestellung. Ein Plädoyer für klare Grenzen* [Child to Order: A Plea for Clear Boundaries], Deutike Verlag, Vienna. Sentences in italics are my comments. Translation by Renate Klein.

107

Canada, England, USA, China and many European countries. They were married couples, homosexuals and single men. Sometimes I receive five emails a day. Some men also send weird messages ... I am very serious when I offer my services. But I don't want a homosexual couple, how can a child grow up without a mother?

Surrogacy is not regulated in Romania. You simply go to a doctor, pay them money and they do it. Or I do it at home. The man gives me his sperm and I put it into my body. No problem. I will pretend to the commissioning couple that I am so pleased I can make a baby for them. I will say that I love being pregnant and I really want to help. They will never know what I really feel. If things are settled between us, I want to go to the doctor with them. In Romania you can fix everything with money. My price is 8,000 euros for the pregnancy and birth. Life is really hard here, prices are high and salaries are low. Surrogacy is a way to earn good money, to have bread on the table. Of course, we do it for the money. That's reasonable, isn't it? It's only the women who need money, or need more of it, who engage in these adventures. It is well-educated, well-paid people who pay us to bear them children, not the other way around. But as a relatively poor woman I have a trump card up my sleeve, I have an advantage. I can do something this rich woman can't do: I can get pregnant. That makes me feel proud. In fact, I feel superior.

There are also many surrogate mothers in Moldova [*a small country between Romania and Ukraine*]. They are poor but healthy, they only eat good food which they produce themselves. They don't smoke, they keep chickens and grow vegetables. It's a good place to find surrogate mothers. There are lots of young women. They are very beautiful. They become surrogate mothers before they go to Italy and become prostitutes. They want between 5,000 and 8,000 euros for a pregnancy and birth. Most of them are already mothers, so they know what will happen.

I've also been thinking about donating eggs but I haven't really looked into it yet. I can do that in Romania too. Of course, commercial egg donation is prohibited but Romania is like the Wild West. The only thing that matters is money, nothing else counts. Our politicians are only interested in how much they earn. And that their corrupt behaviour is not exposed and they don't end up in court.

Left Alone with Exploding Breasts and an Exploding Heart
Michelle (USA)

I have been a surrogate three times. They were all gestational surrogacy (GS) agreements. On each occasion I signed a contract. And I got paid.

One of my surrogacies was a twin pregnancy. Two of my three GS arrangements involved donor eggs. Both sets of parents act as if it is 'no big deal' whether the women who donated the egg ever know of the children that resulted. As far as they're concerned, *possession is nine-tenths of the law.*

I have three children of my own.

My three GS arrangements were brokered out-of-state. There was only one that involved an agency, and the agency stayed around just long enough to collect $5,000 off my uterus, after which I never heard from them again.

I would like to say that I became a surrogate mainly for altruistic reasons. But there were other reasons, and many of them were selfish. I intended to use the money I would make to pay for my education or to put a down payment on a house.

I thought by using a GS surrogacy, maybe there would be no connection with the baby, considering we weren't genetically related. What a sad mistake to make. I now realize it's next to impossible to carry a child without some sense of attachment – and for sure I developed a great deal of attachment.

On each occasion when I was a surrogate there was an enormous amount of pressure. You are locked in by your contract. In fact, in my state, there was no option to change my mind after I had signed. You are absolutely enslaved by the contract.

Throughout each pregnancy, I didn't really receive any money until the end, but there was so much paperwork to ensure I would have almost no legal rights. When money is involved, it's very hard not to feel pressured.

During my first GS, I felt very connected to the baby. I considered taking a train to Michigan to give birth, as I thought that I might be in a more favorable position to fight for custody there. I stopped cashing their checks. They paid me a small monthly allowance; the big check was to come at the end. They were only looking out for their own interests. With my first GS, I didn't even break even. I paid $400+ a month for private health insurance while I was finishing my education. The intending parents never offered to pay the insurance, though they own a $500,000 home, while I own nothing. I later found out the 'Mom' faked a pregnancy so that all her friends and family now believe she carried the child herself. In the meantime she has found it too cumbersome to maintain a relationship with me. She is terrified someone might 'catch us out' if we had lunch together and so discover her secret. Or that her daughter might love her less if she knew the truth.

I had to write into my second and third GS contracts that I would get three hours of 'alone' time with each baby I birthed. This was after my first horrible GS experience. But even then there is really no guarantee. Once the baby is born, you have absolutely no say. You have no contact unless the 'parents' allow it. You are left alone with exploding breasts and an equally exploding sad heart.

I was paid between $18,000 and $35,000 on each occasion. But during all of those pregnancies, I bore costs that the intending parents were contractually obligated to pay. Once the baby or babies are born, it is very hard to collect already paid out monies, or ask extra fees to be paid. The intending parents often literally don't care. I have carried more than one of these children on my health insurance for a time, despite no reimbursement, when legally the fees were not mine to pay.

Before starting the surrogacies, I was advised about potential physical and mental health risks. But I question the process. The fact is that it is difficult, if not impossible, to carry a child for nine months without becoming attached. I have questioned my intending parents' so-called psychological evaluations. In fact, I query whether they actually had any – most don't. If I had known then what I know now about my first GS couple, I never would have carried a baby for them.

I have been very fortunate with my health during all these pregnancies. The biggest problem was the amount of fatigue involved with the twin pregnancy, and the need to stop work at 30 weeks. With the other pregnancies, I worked right up until giving birth.

I had a scare during my current surrogacy with the indication of a triplet pregnancy. My intending mother immediately emailed me saying, "Oh no, please know: if this is a triplet pregnancy, we will reduce." This was very odd, because when I went back through our contract, I found it said the exact opposite, that they would only 'reduce' (that is, abort some of the fetuses) if there was an issue with one of the babies' health. I felt very stuck, not sure what I would do if they insisted on 'reducing' when our contract said otherwise. Fortunately, it never became an issue and I ended up being pregnant with just one baby.

Emotionally, the first GS was the hardest. It still hurts my soul to look back, think about it and write about it. The intending mother had made all sorts of promises before the baby was born, but I had a bad feeling she would not keep them, and I was correct. I had to beg her, "Please let me hold the baby before you leave the room with her. Please." She was not happy about it, but consented – she let me hold the baby before she left the room with her. But I held that baby for less than two minutes. In fact, during my two-day hospital stay, I got to hold that baby for less than five minutes in total. They brought the baby into my room a couple of times. The first time, they said her head was bruised and they didn't want to wake her up, they didn't want her to cry. I took pictures of them by her bassinet. I only got to see the baby.

The second time, they did let me hold her. I held her, she began to stir. I imagine she noticed my presence, and wanted to connect. I put her between my legs on my hospital bed and peeled the blanket back, began peeling back the layers of her clothing. Like any new mom, my instinct was to look at my baby, the one I had carried for more than 40 weeks. As soon as the baby started stirring and making some noise, the intending mother said, "Ah, Ah, Ah!" and reached over to grab her from me, to make sure I didn't see and connect with her any more than I already had. Baby began crying as soon as she was grabbed out of my hands. The intending father then took her out of his partner's hands, stood up, and began talking to her so she would calm down.

I felt very connected to that baby, and I know that baby felt connected to me. I pumped milk for her for eight months. The intending mother had promised me I could drop the milk off each week, hold the baby, and see them both for a while. She broke that promise. Immediately after I went home she emailed me that the intending father would be picking up the milk from my home, and when would be a good time for me? It went on like that for eight months, with me never seeing the baby. I pumped milk five hours a day with a hand-pump and, later, a machine-pump (purchased by me, never once did they offer to pay for, or reimburse me for the time or materials involved in the tedious task of pumping).

They invited me to lunch for the baby's second birthday but I received very poor treatment from 'Mom' there; hatred even. I emailed 'Dad' after I left and let him know I could not, would not, subject myself to that sort of relationship. That if she could not treat me better I needed to end the relationship for my own sake. Dad emailed me back and said I was right to feel that way; Mom had faked a pregnancy and lied to family and friends. She was terrified people would find out she had not carried the baby herself; she was terrified baby would find out she didn't carry her and would love her less. He also said that his wife never plans to tell the baby she was carried by me.

However, instead of allowing me to end our relationship on my terms, his wife dragged it out for another couple of months, inviting me to a BBQ and then to lunch. At the lunch she told me it "wasn't working out." I was mad as hell. I got up and told her to "have a nice life." Why couldn't they let me end our relationship on my terms? But that's her: she must look like she is in control (because in reality she is out of control). She needed to end it in her own, mean, way rather than allowing me to say, "This isn't healthy for me; I must say goodbye."

Right now I feel scared. I'm going to deliver the next baby soon. I hate this feeling of dread. Of not knowing how long I will get to see this kid, if I will get to breastfeed her (I really do want to breastfeed her!), how quickly things will change, how fast I will become irrelevant. People ask me all the time what it's like, and I tell them the honest truth: "It sucks. It's impossible to carry a baby for 40 weeks and not feel any attachment."

I would never, ever advise other women to carry a baby for someone else, whether genetically related or not. Whatever they promise you will not come to fruition. I don't see how a woman can carry a baby and not want to hold it, not want to breastfeed it, not want to change its diapers and whisper loving words in its ear. I actually got 'lucky' with the twin pregnancy I carried, because I did get to do those things. Still, I never see the twins now, and they are not with me. And it is a difficult burden to carry: carrying a little one for that long, having the bond you do, and never knowing what will happen later.

Relinquishing the baby soon after birth is the absolute worst. I think the twin pregnancy felt better for me because I did actually get time with each twin, got to hold them as much as I wanted, got to love them. The singleton was awful. I think the parents thought they were doing themselves a favor by not allowing me to hold her and comfort her. I actually think they set themselves up for a few hard months by not allowing me to hold her, wishing her peace and give me some time. Because that's actually the biggest thing: regardless of how I feel, how do you think that baby feels? People who engage in surrogacy are usually well-educated who know that the baby sees, hears, and smells its environment before she or he is born. And yet they are so willing to snatch it right away from its mother, give it another designation. They are willing to harm a baby just to make sure you don't have any ties to it. It's really disgusting. Babies aren't blank slates. It doesn't matter what are the child's origin, the woman who carried the child has ties to it. To pretend otherwise is just ignorance. You will be hurt. I suggest to every woman who thinks about becoming a surrogate: please consider another way, whether it's for the money, or the delusional idea of self-fulfillment, or whatever. You're not just hurting yourself, you're hurting the baby you carry inside you as well.

A 'Selfless' Donor
Viktoria (Hungary)
As told to Eva Maria Bachinger [6]

Viktoria has blonde hair with dark roots. She wears thick make-up with heavy black kohl around her eyes. This makes her look even paler than she is. Her numerous earrings and bangles jangle as she speaks. She sports many large tattoos. The most noticeable is on her upper arm; it's the face of one of her children. She is now 37 years old and tells me that she is not well. Her menstrual cycle is very irregular, she has frequently recurring headaches, diabetes as well as liver and thyroid problems.

My husband and I went through five IVF cycles so we could have our own child. But it didn't work and we gave up. After that I was hormonally stimulated twice for the purpose of donating eggs. I've never had fertility problems; after all I have four children who are now between eight and 16 years old from an earlier relationship. But after five IVF attempts, I know how painful it is not to be able to have kids when you want them. This is why I decided to donate my eggs. I didn't want any money for it. In Hungary, surplus egg cells are not frozen, so I had to be hormonally stimulated again to produce enough eggs for other women. But the first stimulation almost cost me my life. The doctors told me they harvested 50 egg cells.

---

6   I conducted this interview for my 2015 book *Kind auf Bestellung. Ein Plädoyer für klare Grenzen* [Child to Order: A Plea for Clear Boundaries], Deutike Verlag, Vienna. Sentences in italics are my comments. Translation by Renate Klein.

Ordinarily, far fewer ripe egg cells are harvested, an average of ten. Viktoria's ovary grew to 15 cm when normally an ovary measures 3 to 5 cm.

All I could do was lie on the couch. I couldn't look after my children any more. My belly was hugely distended and very painful. I landed in hospital when water was found in my lungs plus I was told I might get a thrombosis or a lung embolism.

Viktoria had suffered life threatening Ovulation Hyper Stimulation Syndrome (OHSS). But this dangerous wake-up call did not stop her on her mission to be a 'selfless' egg donor for others.

Afterwards, the doctor assured me that this absolutely would not happen again as they would reduce the amount of hormones they injected me with. So I agreed to another stimulation. But unfortunately, I still suffered from adverse effects and felt very ill. The second time I produced 30 egg cells. I felt very proud of myself.

Despite her many health problems since these two procedures and the fact that she is now over 35 – the official age limit for egg donors in Hungary – Viktoria is contemplating embarking on another donation. Officially in Hungary egg donation is only permitted for close relatives. But Viktoria's two donations were for foreigners who she found on the internet.

I received lots of emails and was offered up to 500 euros. Many couples want to keep the egg donation a secret; they do not want their families to know. That's why they do not ask relatives. In Hungary, you have to have a lawyer certify the egg donation contract. When we went to his office, we just said we were all related. He did not check our statements.

For the third egg donation, we – a couple and I – approached an Austrian IVF clinic, because Hungarian IVF centres had already rejected me because of my age. The Austrian clinic offered the procedure to the couple for 15,000 euros. But they thought this was too expensive.

The law in Austria prohibits egg donation for women over 30!

I know that my egg donations led to the birth of two baby girls. Very occasionally I am in touch with their parents. The children don't know that I am their genetic mother. I know that in these babies there are parts of me, but I know that they are not my children. They did not grow in my tummy and I did not give birth to them. They will probably never learn anything about our 'cooperation'! But I find it difficult to remain distant. I was following the progress of both pregnancies with great excitement and occasionally got very worried about the women and their developing babies. I was really pleased when they rang me after visits to the doctor, telling me that everything was fine. I cried with joy when I learnt about the births. It's a fantastic feeling to have been able to help two desperate couples. But it's also weird to see how similar these children are to my own children.

We can only wonder what happened to the more than 70 other egg cells that were 'harvested' from Viktoria. Rumours circulate that there is a lucrative black market for embryos in the Czech Republic. We will never know what happened to Viktoria's eggs.

In her diary Viktoria had noted: "As the day to give birth [for the other woman] draws closer, my desire for a baby produces physical symptoms such as morning sickness. I feel ravaged by emptiness. Each time I see a new mother I experience both jubilation and despair."

I don't regret anything, although I should not have agreed to the second donation. My husband was against it too. I jeopardised my health and I think that it cost me three months of my life because that's how long it took me to feel well again. On the other hand, these families now have a child.

Viktoria excudes the aura of a saint which is in stark contrast to her punk style appearance and large tattoos. Her husband came to our meeting in a café but hardly said a word. As studies show, women often feel guilty for their partner's infertility and seek to compensate for it. But an egg donation is no good deed. It is a serious threat to a woman's health. At the beginning of 2015, Viktoria told me that at a routine health check, a number of cysts and fibroids were found in her womb.

When Good Intentions Were Met with Racism and Hate
Toni (USA)

Deciding to be a surrogate was a spur of the moment decision. My husband and I thought that the only way we could have kids was through IVF because I had had my tubes tied. When I thought about it, I thought ok, maybe we can do surrogacy for another couple first and then they can pay for our IVF cycle? That's why I went the route that I did.

The intended parents and my husband and I were going to go to the same clinic, and it would significantly reduce the amount of money we would have to pay – the IVF was going to cost us only $13,000.

We eventually signed a contract with the intended parents in 2016. My husband and I didn't go through an agency or lawyer, but signed a contract that the intended parents' attorney drew up. I found the intended parents on Craig's List, as crazy as that sounds now. They were advertising for a surrogate on Craig's List and I answered their ad.

The child I carried for them was the genetic child of the intended father, and they used an egg donor, as the intended mother had issues with her own fertility.

I got pregnant on the first embryo transfer. The pregnancy was fine, there were no difficulties. Unfortunately, it only went for six months, but I had gone to all the doctor's appointments and nothing was wrong. There was some bleeding in the beginning that I have heard is common and normal. It was a multiple pregnancy. I was pregnant with twins and so I had a sub-chorionic haemorrhage in the beginning. That's the only thing that happened. Physically everything else was fine.

As soon as we got word that I was pregnant, things started going wrong with the intended parents. I was immediately told that I should be saying "Yes, ma'am" to the intended mother. I was told that my husband could no longer be in the hospital room with me. I was told that I had to get permission if I wanted to go to the hospital if I was bleeding. The intended mother got upset with me because I went to the ER when I was bleeding. That it wasn't my place to decide that. They told me they had hired me – so it was my duty to inform them of everything I wanted to do and I had to get permission from them first.

When it got to that point that she told me I had to start saying "yes, ma'am" to her, she said that she thought I was crazy, because I came from a horrible background. I was really totally floored, because everything had been perfect up to that point. In response, I said at that time I could no longer talk to her and that maybe I needed to talk to the intended father because it was his sperm. But that didn't work either. He was actually the one who said my husband could no longer be in the hospital room with me. At that point I could no longer talk to either of them, and we needed to go through attorneys and we had to go find an attorney. Fortunately, my husband has legal benefits through his job, so the local counsel who helped us in the early days of the case, had his fees covered and we didn't have to pay out of our own pocket.

We dealt with weeks of being harassed while I was pregnant. It got to the point where I didn't feel safe in my own house. When we left our house, we were followed; we had notes left on our cars. My husband had to get a second job to pay for my pregnancy related expenses, like maternity clothes, medical bills, pre-natal vitamins, and my nutritional needs since I was pregnant with twins. Per my contract the intended parents were supposed to pay for those expenses but never did. We had to pay local counsel $2500 and $500 for the *guardian ad litem* filing. They were contacting people in our family. And when I say in our family, I mean even my mother-in-law's ex-husband's daughter. When we went on vacation, somebody tried to break into our house. One of our cars almost blew up of an electrical short. My husband couldn't even make it home from work as a result of this electrical malfunction and he said it looked like the tires had been shredded on the car. It was crazy. Yet even with all that harassment, I was still going to give the babies to them.

What made me decide I could no longer do that was when the intended father sent my sister-in-law a message via Facebook saying that he didn't realize her brother was a dirty f***ing Mexican, and they didn't want him here in this country. And then a couple of days after that she [the intended mother] called me the N-word on the phone.

Unfortunately, I went into pre-term labour at six and a half months. I delivered twin girls by emergency caesarian. They tried to stop the labour but they couldn't. I was only 25 weeks, and the babies were very low birth weight. We lost one eight days later. The other is known as Baby H.

Our case went to the Iowa Supreme Court to seek nonenforcement of the contract to give them the babies. At that time in 2017, the law in Iowa didn't address gestational surrogacy contracts, because technically, we were all committing a Class C felony for selling a human being; for selling a child.

But in 2018 the court ruled that the contract was now enforceable because the judge was sympathetic to people wanting to have their own biological children also stating that I gave up my rights by signing the contract. But the judge ignored parts of our contract, for example, my husband and I were asked to voluntarily give up our rights to Baby H, but we never did do that. I don't know to be honest, I don't know what they're thinking, what they're doing. They now have decided that these kinds of contracts can be enforced in the State of Iowa but the non-biological intended parent has to go through the normal adoption process for the child.

What I don't understand is why the court could enforce part of the contract but not all of it. The Iowa Supreme Court recognised the intended father as the father but told the intended mother she has to go through the adoption process.

My husband and I were called pretty derogatory names by the intended parents as reported widely in the newspapers after the Iowa Supreme Court ruling and after a press briefing in Washington DC. In the court transcripts released was the documentation of these facts as well as the fact the intended parents had been doing background checks on our family members.

We are now asking the US Supreme Court to hear our case, which is being presented in order to challenge the constitutional validity of these contracts. The whole thing has been a nightmare for me and my husband. It has almost destroyed our family.

I would say to anyone who wants to hire a surrogate not to do it. I see a lot of comments in the media and on Facebook by people saying these women knew what they were doing when they signed the contract. You have to understand – I signed a piece of paper before I got pregnant. I signed a piece of paper before I knew the character of these intended parents. After I realized how mean and racist they were, I felt it was my duty to protect these kids from people like that. So you can't say we really knew what we were doing – we only thought we knew what we were doing. But now, we definitely know what we're doing. That's why we're taking the next step to the Supreme Court.

But the whole process is not right. When you marry somebody, you think you're in love with that person. When it doesn't work out, do you have to stay in the marriage? But in surrogacy, we are talking about kids. If in years to come, I would see something bad happening to Baby H if she stays with them, I would never be able to forgive myself for not having tried keeping her.

I think there are plenty of kids out there who can be adopted, I understand that infertile couples want to have their own biological child, but does it really have to be that way? The Court said that Baby

H was not my biological child, but I am still willing and able to fight for her – even if she is not biologically mine. I feel it is my moral duty to protect her. I grew her in my body. I am her birth mother.

What kind of regulations are there to protect Baby H from her intended parents who have behaved so badly? Perhaps such upsetting stories would not happen if intended parents were screened? But lots of people can put on a good face and present themselves as fine upstanding human beings but not be like that in reality.

A lot of people are blaming us surrogates for trying to stop people from making money from surrogacy. Until it happens to you, until you go through something like me or other surrogates out there with their horrific stories, you can't possible imagine how awful it is.

I have now been silenced for almost two years by the courts and I think every day about whether Baby H is going to be okay. The only thing I can do is pray that they're taking care of her and not bring her up in a house full of hate. This wasn't a money or get-rich-quick type of scheme. If that were the case, I would have wanted to be paid more than $13,000. We just wanted enough money for one cycle of IVF so that we could have our own child, and still to this day, they never even paid me one dollar.

I think surrogacy should be stopped.

That's where I stand now. If you are thinking about being a surrogate, I understand your heart might be in a good place. But I tell you, it's not worth the chance of going through what I and so many others that I have found out since, have gone through. It's not worth it. And then you involve these innocent babies in your fights.

The intended parents have tried to drag my name through the mud. But I am strong. Now that I can speak out I will be attacked, but whatever criticism I cop won't be as bad as what they have said about me already.

I know why I did what I did and the reason for doing it. But now I will keep standing up and continue to fight for Baby H.

Note: In October 2018, the U.S. Supreme Court denied the petition to review this case. That means that the Iowa Supreme Court ruling that surrogacy contracts are enforceable will stand and Baby H will remain with the intended parents.

Afterword

As we were working with our contributors on this book, there were daily updates on the state of surrogacy around the world. On the one hand, a growing number of governments in Asia such as Thailand, India, Nepal and Cambodia wisely closed their doors to surrogacy. Indications are that Ireland will follow soon. France, Germany, Sweden and Switzerland stand firm in their rejection of surrogacy. As well, the European Parliament has repeatedly condemned surrogacy. Some countries, like Australia and the UK, only allow so-called altruistic surrogacy. In the USA, ten states have explicitly legalised commercial surrogacy. The vast majority of countries in the world prohibit surrogacy.

On the other hand, ignoring ethical and human rights concerns, the surrogacy industry forges ahead with new global fertility enterprises, especially in Eastern Europe (Ukraine, Georgia and Russia) and also in Greece and Cyprus where poor women abound.

But fortunately, we are witnessing growing resistance. Since May 2015 we have a global movement: *Stop Surrogacy Now* (stopsurrogacynow.com) with more than 10,000 signatories. In France in 2018, a Coalition for the Abolition of Surrogate Motherhood (ICASM) was founded, and in Spain, in 2018, the International Campaign for a Global Ban on Womb Rental gathered hundreds of signatures from feminist groups and individuals around the world.

Contrary to what the promoters of surrogacy claim, more and more concerned individuals and groups are beginning to push back against the exploitation of women and children in this industry.

No doubt the heartbreaking story of Baby Gammy changed many minds. The little boy with Down syndrome born to 'surrogate' mother Pattaramon Chanbua in Thailand captivated the world after his commissioning parents left Thailand with his unaffected twin sister Pipah. The fact that their intended father had been previously jailed for child sex offences in Australia also caused outrage.

Australian Chief Justice of the Family Court, Judge Pascoe, said that in his view, surrogacy is "likely to expose vulnerable women and children to terrible abuse." He believes that the Gammy case

> highlights the plight of surrogate mothers and unwanted commissioned children ... the scandal is accentuated by the commissioning parent being a convicted paedophile, which potentially exposes the children to danger. The most basic of background checks on the father is glaringly absent. ... The international commercial surrogacy market can, and is, being used by people ill-suited to be parents (Pascoe 2014).

Indeed, horror stories abound. Australian Peter Truong and his American partner Mark Newton bought a baby boy from a Russian 'surrogate' mother specifically to abuse and sell in international paedophile rings (Klein, 2017; Meldrum-Hanna and Masters 2018). Alas, this was not an isolated case. In 2016, a commissioning father who trafficked and sexually abused surrogate twin baby daughters in Australia was sentenced to 22 years imprisonment after pleading guilty to 37 charges including 20 counts of incest and two of child trafficking (Australian Broadcasting Corporation 2016).

These cases undermine the surrogacy industry's legitimacy and threaten its business. In response, surrogacy promoters maintain 'regulation' is the answer. But regulation will never work. A multitude of laws throughout the world only wait for one thing: to be broken.

Furthermore, regulation actually *reinforces* the practice of surrogacy. In its refusal to go to the *roots* of surrogacy and expose it for what it is – the trafficking and buying of babies as commodities, the human rights violation of 'surrogate' mothers and egg 'donors' – it tinkers around the edges of what should be allowed, how 'parentage' should be legislated (as the Hague Conference on Private

International Law, HCCH, is currently undertaking in its Parentage/ Surrogacy Project).[7]

Surrogacy contracts underline the fallacy of regulation. They are invariably based on inequality between the 'buyers' – financially superior intended parents, both hetero- and homosexual – and the sellers – economically disadvantaged women as so-called surrogates and egg providers, often also belonging to a marginalised ethnicity, class or caste.

Many contributors to this book undertook surrogacy within a contractual agreement. It is glaringly obvious that these contracts exist primarily to protect the interests of the commissioning parents, not the woman. The whole point of the contract is to *control* the 'surrogate' mother for the nine months of the pregnancy. This 'management' ignores best practice in maternal healthcare, and in many cases contradicts it (Mbadiwe 2018).

For the Eastern European and Indian women represented in *Broken Bonds*, surrogacy contracts severely curtailed their personal autonomy. They gave up their freedom to earn money for their families. This is nothing less than abuse of poor women. Sheela Saravanan's 2018 book *A Transnational Feminist View of Surrogacy Biomarkets in India* portrays the heartbreaking reality of the desperate poverty in which many Indian women live with their children, and the conditions they endure in surrogacy arrangements simply to provide for their families.

And how does the wealthy West compare? We certainly exploit women and babies in a more sanitised manner. In California, the most surrogacy-friendly place in the world, and other US states such as Oregon, surrogacy contracts ensure that the intended parents will be the legal parents of the child. Some of them do this with a pre-birth certificate. The 'surrogate' mother cannot change her mind and keep the child. She is in fact never referred to as a 'mother' of any

---

7   For a detailed discussion on the regulation of surrogacy including HCCH and why it will never work, see Chapter 5 of Renate Klein's 2017 book *Surrogacy: A Human Rights Violation*.

kind. She is a 'gestational surrogate'. A carrier. For a gay male couple or a single man commissioning a baby via surrogacy, there is no legal mother.

The commissioning parents control the 'surrogate' mother's food selection, her exercise and travel, living arrangements and intimate relationships. They have access to her medical records and determine if she should abort the pregnancy or not (in the case of suspected abnormality or multiple foetuses). One contract stipulates, "The Surrogate and her Husband agree that they will neither form, nor attempt to form, a parent-child relationship with any Child the surrogate may bear," in an overt attempt to prohibit maternal-infant bonding.

Extra-contractual demands have to be followed under the threat of not getting paid. Thus many commissioning parents and clinics are able to act contrary to the contracts with impunity. Regulation always works in favour of those with the money and the power. This is inevitable. This is what regulation is intended to do in the first place.

Regulation of surrogacy necessarily requires that the woman must sign away her right to privacy, doctor/patient confidentiality, bodily integrity, medical decision-making power, and more. It is unacceptable that anyone loses these rights, even if only for a specified time. The child, of course, has no say in the matter – she or he will become permanently separated from the birth mother in these transactions. If we took into account the 'best interests of the child' as well as women's right to integrity of body and soul, surrogacy would never happen at all.

A look at some United Nations Conventions and other international instruments confirm our position:[8]

The United Nations Slavery Convention: Article 1 of the Convention of September 26, 1926 concerning slavery defines slavery as "the status or condition of a person over whom any or

---

8   See the 2015 Draft Convention for the Abolition of Surrogacy by CoRP <https://collectif-corp.com/2015/03/24/hague-conference-feminists-for-the-abolition-of-surrogacy/>

all of the powers attaching to the right of ownership are exercised." There is no doubt that surrogacy closely resembles a modern form of slavery according to this definition.

The International Convention on the Rights of the Child: Article 7 §1 of this Convention stipulates, "The child shall be registered immediately after birth and shall have the right from birth to a name, the right to acquire a nationality and as far as possible, the right to know and be cared for by his or her parents. "

Surrogacy thus clearly violates Article 7 §1 of the Convention on the Rights of the Child.

The Convention on the Elimination of All Forms of Discrimination Against Women (CEDAW): Article 3 of this Convention stipulates that "States Parties shall take in all fields, in particular in the political, social, economic and cultural fields, all appropriate measures, including legislation, to ensure the full development and advancement of women, for the purpose of guaranteeing them the exercise and enjoyment of human rights and fundamental freedoms on a basis of equality with men." As CoRP *et al.* comment:

> The practice of surrogacy involves appropriating in a specific manner the reproductive capacities of women. It leads to the implementation of an extremely firm control over every aspect of women's lives during pregnancy and endangers their physical and psychological health in order to satisfy the desires of sponsoring third parties.
>
> In this sense, the practice is profoundly discriminatory and is contrary to the objective of the full development of women and of progress towards women's full enjoyment of their fundamental human rights.

There are other International Agreements that can be invoked. They all show convincingly that surrogacy is a profoundly illegal activity. And yet, clinics and agencies lure people desperate for a child of their own with carefully crafted advertising and selective information. They go to great lengths to protect the image of surrogacy and hide its illegitimacy. And of course a lucrative industry with such desperate customers always attracts criminal elements. Theresa Ericson, a

California-based surrogacy attorney who was convicted and sent to prison for leading a baby-selling ring, called herself the "tip of the iceberg, when it comes to people abusing the system" (Lahl 2018).

We must defy pro-surrogacy consumer groups such as *Families through Surrogacy* in Australia, or the US group *Men Having Babies*. Casting a look over their corporate sponsors and 'partners', the enormous vested global interests in surrogacy advocacy comes to light. This is where the money really goes.

Those contemplating the option of surrogacy as a means of having children need to be aware that behind the slick marketing and glossy publicity of intermediaries motivated by profit, are the traumatic consequences for the women who are made invisible by this industry: the women who give birth to children they often never see again.

In documenting just some of the many stories of heartbreak around the lived experiences of being birth mothers and egg providers, *Broken Bonds* shows that human rights violations are inherent in this practice. Surrogacy is not just a means of having children but necessitates *harming* women and children; children who may never know the woman who gave birth to them. The concept of ethical surrogacy is a myth, a myth that disguises the power imbalances between participants (see Klein, 2017).

Our natural instinct is to welcome and celebrate the arrival of all children. But the wallpapering of surrogacy stories with gurgling babies has contributed to a reluctance to critique the profit-driven industry which has thrived mostly unchallenged by ethical analysis or close scrutiny of its questionable practices.

Broken Bonds is one small step towards exposing Big Fertility operations by giving voice to those harmed by them. We sincerely hope that these brave voices will be heard and heeded and that people considering embarking on surrogacy will change their mind.

Surrogacy is a blatant abuse of the rights of women and children. But it is not inevitable. It can be stopped. Join the growing global movement of *Stop Surrogacy Now* at www.stopsurrogacy.com and sign the statement below.

Stop Surrogacy Now Statement

We are women and men of diverse ethnic, religious, cultural, and socio-economic backgrounds from all regions of the world. We come together to voice our shared concern for women and children who are exploited through surrogacy contract pregnancy arrangements.

Together we affirm the deep longing that many have to be parents. Yet, as with most desires, there must be limits. Human rights provide an important marker for identifying what those limits should be. We believe that surrogacy should be stopped because it is an abuse of women's and children's human rights.

Surrogacy often depends on the exploitation of poorer women. In many cases, it is the poor who have to sell and the rich who can afford to buy. These unequal transactions result in consent that is under-informed if not uninformed, low payment, coercion, poor health care, and severe risks to the short- and long-term health of women who carry surrogate pregnancies.

The medical process for surrogacy entails risks for the surrogate mother, the young women who sell their eggs, and the children born via the assisted reproductive technologies employed. The risks to women include Ovarian Hyper Stimulation Syndrome (OHSS), ovarian torsion, ovarian cysts, chronic pelvic pain, premature menopause, loss of fertility, reproductive cancers, blood clots, kidney disease, stroke, and, in some cases, death. Women who become pregnant with eggs from another woman are at higher risk for pre-eclampsia and high blood pressure.

Children born of assisted reproductive technologies, which are usually employed in surrogacy, also face known health risks that include: preterm birth, stillbirth, low birth weight, fetal anomalies, and higher blood pressure. A surrogate pregnancy intentionally severs the natural maternal bonding that takes places in pregnancy – a bond that medical professionals consistently encourage and promote. The biological link between mother and child is undeniably intimate, and when severed has lasting repercussions felt by both. In places where surrogacy is legalized, this potential harm is institutionalized.

We believe that the practice of commercial surrogacy is indistinguishable from the buying and selling of children. Even when non-commercial (that is, unpaid or "altruistic"), any practice that subjects women and children to such risks must be banned.

No one has a right to a child, whether they are heterosexual, homosexual, or single-by-choice.

We stand together asking national governments of the world and leaders of the international community to work together to end this practice and **Stop Surrogacy Now**.

Acknowledgements

Jennifer Lahl

I am deeply grateful for all the women who have entrusted me with their most intimate stories of harm, abuse, and feelings of hopelessness. I can only imagine the personal cost to you; loss of privacy, damaged health, financial ruin, and the stress on your own families, as you have bravely come forward to tell your story in order to protect others.

You know first hand that those who needed your body, profited off your body, want nothing more than to silence or discredit you. I am sorry that the fertility industry has allowed this to happen to you and I promise to always defend and advocate for you. And to keep telling your powerful and important stories until the necessary changes occur.

To my partners in this project, Renate and Melinda, while we've never even met, we have worked together for so long that I count each of you as dear friends in this battle to demand justice. It's sad that such causes have brought us together, but until the wrongs of the world are righted, it is an honor and privilege to labor (hopefully, not in vain) alongside each of you. My heart leapt for joy when you both asked me to be a part of this book!

Pauline and Susan, how do you do it? Your organizational skills have yet to meet their match. Thank you for keeping us all on task and keeping track of all the details that go into a collective project such as *Broken Bonds*.

To Dan, who always cheers me on and believes in me more than I often believe in myself.

Melinda Tankard Reist

The women who contributed to this book must be acknowledged first. Without them, *Broken Bonds* would not exist. We are so grateful to you for sharing your experiences with us and honour you, your enduring love for the children you carried and birthed and for desiring to warn other women so that they may not become fodder in this voracious global industry.

Renate – to have my name alongside yours on a book cover – well that's something I couldn't have dreamed of when we first met (25?) years ago in Bangladesh. Your pioneering writing on reproductive technologies first introduced me to feminist bioethics. And now, here we are ...

Jennifer – your work exposing the harms of *Big Fertility* has been at the vanguard of the global movement against it. Thank you for caring for all the women harmed by this industry and, through the Center for Bioethics and Culture, providing a place for the injustice they have suffered to be heard and acknowledged.

Selena – thanks for being my right arm in this project. I couldn't have done it without you.

Pauline – for going above and beyond to make this book happen.

And thank you Susan – for always valuable advice and input and for being a steadying influence on all of us! To Spinifex for believing in my ideas and publishing them. I am grateful for our partnership and for the five books we have created together.

To family and friends for sharing burdens and lightening loads.

Renate Klein

Like Jennifer and Melinda, my biggest thank you goes to the women – and one man – who have entrusted us with their infuriating experiences in the surrogacy industry. And to Eva Maria Bachinger and Sheela Saravanan for your path breaking work: soul sisters. In my more than 30 years as a critic of reproductive technologies including surrogacy, I have always believed that if people only knew what really goes on in this industry and how much women are harmed, lied to and harassed, they would join forces with us trying to put an end to Big Fertility Inc.

I fervently hope that *Broken Bonds* will change minds. No better friends than Jennifer and Melinda to work on this book, not always in easy circumstances when we are geographically separated and overworked: Thank you both for your continuing work to make the world a better place for women and girls (and yes Melinda it has been 25 years since we first met). I look forward to that celebratory drink when we finally all get together!

Thank you also to Selena Ewing for your valuable input to this project. It was a pleasure working with you.

The Spinifex Team has been as marvellous as always. Thank you to Deb Snibson for the awesome cover and to Susan Hawthorne for never losing your cool. Pauline Hopkins deserves a whole bucket of gold stars: without your firm hands this book would not have come together. But I also want to acknowledge your outstanding editing work on the two Australian stories and thank you for your dedication. And you are a pleasure to work with as well.

All of us involved in this project have been in tears. In tears of rage, of anger, of disbelief about how the surrogacy industry players mistreat women. In tears because we felt so frustrated about what the women writing in this book had to endure. May *Broken Bonds* sound a clarion call to the world to put an end to this abuse.

Pleasant Hill, Canberra and Mission Beach
December 2018

References

ABC News (20 February 2018). 'Thai court grants 28-year-old Japanese man custody of 13 surrogate children'. *ABC Online;* <http://www.abc.net.au/news/2018-02-20/japanese-man-granted-paternity-rights-to-13-surrogate-children/9467790>

Azhar, Mian (30 November 2018). 'Five Ways to Know if You'd Make a Good Gestational Surrogate'. *The Good Men Project;* <https://goodmenproject.com/parenting/five-ways-to-know-if-youd-make-a-good-gestational-surrogate/>

Bindel, Julie (16 September 2016). 'The selling of subordination: How the female body is reduced to products'. *Truthdig;* <https://www.truthdig.com/articles/the-selling-of-subordination-how-the-female-body-is-reduced-to-products/>

Bray, Abigail (2013). *Misogyny Re-Loaded.* Spinifex Press, North Melbourne.

CBC Network (2018). *#Big Fertility: It's All About the Money.* <https://vimeo.com/ondemand/bigfertility/289386333>

Cottingham Jane (2017). 'Babies, Borders and Big Business'. *Reproductive Health Matters* 25(49):17-20; <https://www.tandfonline.com/doi/pdf/10.1080/09688080.2017.1360603>

Donor Conception Support Group of Australia (1997). *Let the Offspring Speak: Discussions on Donor Conception.* Georges Hall, New South Wales.

Du Cann, Gerard and Sofia Petkar, (29 September 2018). 'Man finds out his biological dad is a 'super sperm donor' and that he could have 1,000 siblings – and now he wants to find them ALL'. *The Sun;* <https://www.thesun.co.uk/news/7378145/man-finds-biological-dad-super-sperm-donor-1000-siblings/>

Ekman Ekis, Kajsa (2013). *Being and Being Bought: Prostitution, Surrogacy and the Split Self.* Spinifex Press, North Melbourne.

Hurst, Daniel (20 February 2018). 'Japanese man wins sole custody of 13 surrogacy children'. *The Guardian;* <https://www.theguardian.com/world/2018/feb/20/japanese-man-custody-13-surrogate-children-thai-court>

Kane, Elizabeth (1988/90). *Birth Mother: The Story of America's First Legal Surrogate Mother.* Harcourt, San Diego; Sun Books, Macmillan, South Melbourne.

Klein, Renate (2008). 'From test-tube women to bodies without women'. *Women's Studies International Forum* 31(3):157-75. <https://www.sciencedirect.com/science/article/abs/pii/S0277539508000290>

Klein, Renate (2017). *Surrogacy: A Human Rights Violation.* Spinifex Press, North Melbourne.

Kuczynski, Alex (28 November 2008). 'Her body, my baby'. *The New York Times Magazine;* <https://www.nytimes.com/2008/11/30/magazine/30Surrogate-t.html>

Lahl, Jennifer (15 April 2018). 'Surrogacy: no laughing matter'. *Public Discourse: The Journal of the Witherspoon Institute*; <https://www.thepublicdiscourse. com/2018/04/21343/>

Lee-St John, Jeninne (13 December 2007). 'The 10 best chores to outsource'. *Time Magazine*; <http://content.time.com/time/magazine/article/ 0,9171,1694454,00.html>

Lorbach, Caroline (2003). *Experiences of Donor Conception: Parents, Offspring and Donors through the Years*. Jessica Kingsley Publishers, London.

Lynch, Catherine (2018). Submission to the Western Australian Review of the Human Reproductive Technology Act 1991 and the Surrogacy Act 2008.

MacDonald, Sarah (4 August 2014). 'What Baby Gammy's story teaches us about commercial surrogacy'. *Daily Life;* <http://www.dailylife.com.au/life-and-love/parenting-and-families/what-baby-gammys-story-teaches-us-about-commercial-surrogacy-20140804-3d4ac>

Mbadiwe, Tafari (9 October 2018). 'Mistaking legal recourse for evidence-based medical practices in surrogacy'. *Medical Bag;* <https://www.medicalbag.com/ medicine/surrogate-pregnancy-legal-medical-challenges/article/805954/>

Meldrum-Hanna, Caro and Deb Masters (26 February 2018). 'Boy with henna tattoo: How Australian Peter Truong groomed son to be exploited by global paedophile network'. *Australian Broadcasting Corporation;* <https://www.abc. net.au/news/2014-03-10/boy-with-henna-tattoo-network-exposed/5310812>

New South Wales Government, Animal Welfare Branch, Industry and Investment. (2009). *Animal Welfare Code of Practice: Breeding Dogs and Cats.* <https://www. dpi.nsw.gov.au/__data/assets/pdf_file/0004/299803/Breeding-dogs-and-cats-code-of-practice.pdf>

Norma, Caroline and Tankard Reist, Melinda (2016). *Prostitution Narratives: Stories of Survival in the Sex Trade.* Spinifex Press, North Melbourne.

Pascoe, John (2014). 'Parenting and Children's Issues: International Commercial Surrogacy and the risk of abuse'. *3rd Annual LegalWise International Family Law Conference,* Shanghai, China, 17-20 September 2014. <http://www.abc.net.au/ reslib/201409/r1332410_18536962.pdf>

Raymond, Janice (1996). 'Connecting Reproductive and Sexual Liberalism'. In Diane Bell and Renate Klein (eds) *Radically Speaking: Feminism Reclaimed.* Spinifex Press, North Melbourne, pp. 231-246.

Récamier-Corballo, Soledad, Erika Estrada-Camarena and Caroline López-Rubalcava (2018). 'Maternal separation induces long term effects on monoamines and brain-derived neurotrophic factor levels on the frontal cortex, amygdala, and hippocampus: differential effects after a stress challenge'. *Behavioural Pharmacology* 28(7), pp. 545–557.

Riben, Mirah (30 May 2015). 'Human Factory Farming and the Campaign to Outlaw Surrogacy'. *Dissident Voice;* <https://dissidentvoice.org/2015/05/human-factory-farming-and-the-campaign-to-outlaw-surrogacy/#more-58594>

Saravanam, Sheela (2018). *A Transnational Feminist View of Surrogacy Biomarkets in India.* Springer, Singapore.

Smith, Kyle (3 October 2013). 'Pregnancy got you down? No problem, outsource your babymaking to India'. *Forbes Magazine;* <https://www.forbes.com/sites/

kylesmith/2013/10/03/pregnancy-got-you-down-no-problem-outsource-your-babymaking-to-india/#7f5be656fb49>

Surrogate.com. 'How to emotionally transfer a baby born via surrogacy'. <https://surrogate.com/intended-parents/raising-a-child-born-from-surrogacy/how-to-emotionally-transfer-a-baby-born-via-surrogacy/>

Tankard Reist, Melinda (ed) (2006). *Defiant Birth: Women Who Resist Medical Eugenics.* Spinifex Press, North Melbourne.

Thaivisa.com (24 February 2011). 'Thai police free women from illegal baby farm in Bangkok'; <https://www.thaivisa.com/forum/topic/446023-thai-police-free-women-from-illegal-baby-farm-in-bangkok/>

Tremblay, Joey (28 November 2018). '"Who's the mother?" Two new dads embrace parenthood after surrogate birth.' *CBC News;* <https://www.cbc.ca/news/canada/saskatchewan/surrogate-new-dads-baby-born-regina-1.4922384>

Verrier, Nancy (1996). *The Primal Wound: Understanding the Adopted Child.* Gateway Press, Baltimore MD.

Victoria State Government (2018). *Code of Practice for the Private Keeping of Cats.* Victoria.

Whitelocks, Sadie (5 December 2016). '"I don't want to give up the baby": Surrogate mothers confess how they REALLY feel about carrying someone else's child.' *Daily Mail UK;* <https://www.dailymail.co.uk/femail/article-3982896/Surrogate-mothers-tell-Whisper-website-feels-carry-s-child.html>

Winston, Robert (11 July 2018). 'IVF 'gravy train' giving couples false hope says senior medic Prof Robert Winston.' *The Irish Times;* <https://www.irishnews.com/lifestyle/2018/07/12/news/professor-robert-winston-couples-being-misled-about-the-dream-of-ivf-treatment-1378545/>

Wollstonecraft, Mary (1792). *A Vindication of the Rights of Woman.* Thomas and Andrews, Boston.

Woo, Irene, Rita Hindoyan, Melanie Landay, Jacqueline Ho, Sue Ann Ingles, Lynda McGinnis, Richard Paulson and Karine Chung (2017). 'Perinatal outcomes after natural conception versus in vitro fertilization (IVF) in gestational surrogates: a model to evaluate IVF treatment versus maternal effects.' *Fertility and Sterility* 108 (6), pp. 993–998.

Other books available from Spinifex Press

Surrogacy: A Human Rights Violation
Renate Klein

Pared down to cold hard facts, surrogacy is the commissioning/ buying/renting of a woman into whose womb an embryo is inserted and who thus becomes a 'breeder' for a third party.

In *Surrogacy: A Human Rights Violation* Renate Klein details her objections to surrogacy by examining the short- and long-term harms done to the so-called surrogate mothers, egg providers and the female partner in a heterosexual commissioning couple. The author also looks at the rights of children and compares surrogacy to (forced) adoption practices. She concludes that surrogacy, whether so-called altruistic or commercial, can never be ethical and she outlines forms of resistance to stop surrogacy.

ISBN 9781925581034 | AUD $19.95 | eBook available

Being and Being Bought: Prostitution, Surrogacy and the Split Self
Kajsa Ekis Ekman

Kajsa Ekis Ekman argues that in prostitution the Self must be split from the body to make it possible to sell your body without selling yourself. The body becomes sex. Sex becomes a service.

Turning to the practice of surrogate motherhood, Kajsa Ekis Ekman identifies the same components: that the woman is forced to disconnect from her own body and to the child she gives birth to. The product sold is not sex but a baby. Ekis Ekman asks: why should this not be called child trafficking?

This brilliant exposé is written with a razor-sharp intellect and disarming wit and will make us look at prostitution and surrogacy and the parallels between them in a new way.

ISBN: 9781742198767 | AUD $29.95 | eBook available

*If you would like to know more about
Spinifex Press, write to us for a free catalogue, visit our
website or email us for further information
on how to subscribe to our monthly newsletter.*

Spinifex Press
PO Box 105
Mission Beach QLD 4852
Australia

www.spinifexpress.com.au
women@spinifexpress.com.au